THE BLEEP TEST

What does it mean to help save someone's life? How does it feel to nearly kill a patient? Can we keep our patients safe at night? In the face of overwhelming pressures, can we thrive or only survive? And is a happy life as a doctor still possible?

In the early months and years of work, it is these kinds of questions, rather than any technical or knowledge-based queries, which preoccupy many new doctors. This elusive, hidden curriculum is pervasive within departments, around hospitals and across health systems, but is rarely, if ever, explicitly examined and discussed. At its core is the issue that should matter above all others – how we can keep our patients as safe as possible.

The Bleep Test combines gripping and startlingly vulnerable recollections of early experiences on the wards with an array of research findings, from psychology and human biology to anthropology, business and behavioural economics. Acknowledging that the truly complex challenges facing new doctors lie far beyond the realms of the traditional medical sciences in which they were trained, the book explains that the shift to being a doctor depends on first understanding how we think, reason and behave as someone we have been all our lives – a human amongst humans.

Focused on the experiences of, and the issues facing, recently qualified medics, *The Bleep Test* is not only for young doctors but also for anyone who manages them, works with them, cares for them or may one day depend on them.

THE BLEEP TEST

How New Doctors Can Get Things Right

Luke Austen BM BCh, MRCP(UK)

CRC Press
Taylor & Francis Group
Boca Raton London

CRC Press is an imprint of the
Taylor & Francis Group, an **informa** business

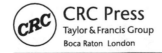

First edition published 2023
by CRC Press
6000 Broken Sound Parkway NW, Suite 300, Boca Raton, FL 33487–2742

and by CRC Press
4 Park Square, Milton Park, Abingdon, Oxon, OX14 4RN

CRC Press is an imprint of Taylor & Francis Group, LLC

ISBN: 978-1-032-42237-4 (hbk)
ISBN: 978-1-032-41490-4 (pbk)
ISBN: 978-1-003-36188-6 (ebk)

DOI: 10.1201/9781003361886

Typeset in Joanna
by Apex CoVantage, LLC

CONTENTS

FOREWORD

The training of medical students is always an ongoing discussion necessitating changes in the curriculum every few years to keep up with progress. We have got away from the didactic teaching of yesteryear to a more focused approach on students and how they learn. Ultimately, of course, it is how they approach and speak to the patient. This skill is taught initially in clinical laboratories, by learning methodologies, single patient encounters, and then onto wards, clinics, or GP surgeries, where students will practise their newly acquired skills on patients. These measures may lessen the anxiety of that first patient encounter, but the student does this in the quiet surroundings of a ward and is closely supervised. Nothing, however, lessens that overnight transformation from a student with little responsibility, to being the doctor responsible for someone else's life. A huge leap into the unknown!

In a Lancet editorial in 1999, Chandler said that "medicine used to be simple, ineffective and safe; now it is complex, effective but relatively dangerous." How very true but, of course, this adds to the anxiety of suddenly becoming a 'doctor' and the dawning realisation that now is the 'real thing' that one has striven for, over at least 5–6 years. With the development of many new therapies, devices, and drugs, a physician is now faced with an armamentarium of therapies all of which need to be carefully considered, with their side effects, cross reactions, and toxicity, prior to prescribing. All adding to stress and anxiety.

So, how does one approach this massive 'leap to responsibility'? Will 'The Bleep Test' help?

I started reading this book thinking it would contain a long list of things that a new doctor might, or should, do. I was therefore taken aback when it was more about the person and the thoughts and feelings that the new doctor encountered. The incidents and events are descriptions of real-life encounters. The book tackles the first few years of being a doctor relating real experiences but with a background account of self-reflective thoughts that went through the author's mind. It is semi-autobiographical and therefore more authentic. For example, the author describes the multi-tasking, frenetic and anxious junior doctor switching between problems with lists of 'to do' jobs and the difficulty they had with prioritising. I remember doing this myself when my junior doctor asked me to swap places with her as she thought consultants didn't have much to do! Despite my many years of experience as a consultant, I found that prioritising patients' problems was the most difficult, particularly when one's 'to do' list was thrown out of kilter, as a crash call came in for someone with very severe chest pain.

The author goes through the emotions he encountered. Emotions of fright, when confronted with a difficult problem, anxiety when not knowing what to do, and embarrassment when your indecision to act led to a ward clerk correctly calling for help for a patient who 'didn't look well'! Experience is clearly key but so is an insight into yourself. This is particularly true when owning up to (and learning from) a mistake you had made in giving the wrong drug to a patient with incomplete knowledge because you had not taken a full history.

'The Bleep Test' is easy to read and almost like a novel. It is scattered with useful diagrams and very well referenced. There are many other similar books on the market but none quite like this one. This explores the mind and emotions triggered off by clinical situations. This is an important pointer to all of us when we try and understand the very high incidence of burnout and mental health problems in the profession. I would certainly recommend this book to all young doctors but also to medical students to give them an understanding of what is ahead for them. Senior doctors should read this to remember what they went through themselves, making them even more understanding and supportive to their juniors. The book is written without medical jargon and therefore would be of great interest to the general public for an insight into our profession. It might help them appreciate what emotions a caring professional must go through to be able to improve the health of the population.

Professor Dame Parveen Kumar DBE
Emerita Professor of Medicine and Education
Barts and the London School of Medicine and Dentistry,
Queen Mary University of London

AUTHOR'S NOTE

All of the stories in this book have a basis in my own and my colleagues' clinical experiences, but in order to protect patient confidentiality numerous identifying details such as name, sex, ethnicity and medical problems have been changed or merged so as to be unrecognisable. Any similarities to real people are therefore coincidental.

MEDICAL LANGUAGE AND AMERICAN SPELLING

Although *The Bleep Test* is written first and foremost for new doctors, I hope that others, even non-medically trained, may also find it interesting or useful. I have therefore tried to keep technical medical language to a minimum, but inevitably it does crop up in places. If you find yourself having to search a few terms online here and there, I'm sure that your tablet or smartphone will ping you an explanation much faster than you could flick through to a glossary.

Doctors do, however, have a love for TLAs (three-letter acronyms). I am no exception, so a list of the ones in this book is included at the end.

The spelling and terminology used in the book are British, but where the research or source in question has come from the United States, I haven't altered it. For example, in Chapter 3 we hear about 'anesthesiology residents' rather than 'anaesthetics trainees'.

INTRODUCTION

BLACK WEDNESDAY

At 20 minutes to 8 on the evening of Wednesday 16 September 1992, the Chancellor of the Exchequer Norman Lamont emerged from the Treasury to face the music. A crisis of confidence in the pound sterling had led to a run on the currency that the Bank of England had been unable to reverse. Lamont was forced to admit defeat and announce that the pound would fall out of the European Exchange Rate Mechanism. It was the culmination of a day from which his government would never truly recover; it became known as 'Black Wednesday'.

These kinds of days of reckoning for the British economy are (we hope) a rarity. But every year the nation faces a 'Black Wednesday' crisis of confidence of a different kind. The first Wednesday of August is the day when recently graduated medical students set foot on the wards as qualified doctors for the first time, finally after years of training being handed some responsibility for patient care. And almost 26 years after Lamont's concession, I was one of them. We were mostly enthusiastic and keen to get started, but it was an anxious and nervy moment. Medical school was finished, and whilst all junior doctors are 'doctors in training', we were no longer in the hospital purely for our own education. The stakes were higher, and we knew it.

In 2009, Min Hua Jen and colleagues published a study titled "Early In-Hospital Mortality Following Trainee Doctors' First Day at Work", reporting that the odds of dying within seven days of admission for patients admitted as an emergency on the first Wednesday of August were 6% higher than for patients admitted on the last Wednesday of July.[1] The group retrospectively analysed data from the previous nine years, investigating just under 300,000 emergency admissions and uncovering this worrying variation in outcomes for people apparently unlucky enough to fall ill right when hospitals were taking on inexperienced new starters.

Although the increase in mortality was statistically significant, Abi Rimmer pointed out in the *BMJ* that the absolute number of deaths in the study was low, amounting to only 45 excess Black Wednesday deaths over a period of nine years.[2] In response to her article, three of my medical school colleagues found from a freedom of information request to a single NHS trust that consultants in specialties including anaesthetics, emergency medicine and oncology had taken significantly more days of annual leave in August compared with June, presumably due to school holidays.[3] They suggested that the availability of consultant expertise might also be an important factor behind any increase in August mortality. What's more, Jen and colleagues themselves concluded that they could not determine any causal link between the arrival of new junior doctors and the higher mortality rates, and that further work would be necessary to evaluate if any of the excess deaths were preventable. However, the idea of it all was enough. The newspapers had a field day, and the concept of Black Wednesday for the NHS went mainstream.

The notion of higher mortality rates coinciding with new doctors starting work was not a new one, with debates about the existence of a Black Wednesday effect stretching back nearly three decades. A character in Jed Mercurio's BBC drama *Cardiac Arrest* stating, "You come out of medical school knowing bugger all – no wonder August is the killing season"[4] prompted a 1994 study published in the *BMJ* that did not find any evidence that hospital patients were more likely to die in the first week of August than at other times of the year,[5] although that study was not of comparable quality to Jen's later work.

In the United States, the issue is referred to as the 'July effect', since first-year residents (interns) arrive on the wards one month ahead of their British counterparts. It has been investigated extensively on both sides of the Atlantic with various studies supporting or refuting its existence, alongside many papers offering solutions to mitigate the potential impending harm. Bob Wachter, Professor and Chair of the Department of Medicine at the University of California, San Francisco, spoke about the July effect on the *Freakonomics MD* podcast. He mused:

> It's not 100% clear there is such a thing. You can find studies that support that the July effect is real. You can find studies that find not much effect. But I say, when you look at the studies . . . you come away with the general feeling that, if you had to put your nickel down, you would say there is a July effect.[6]

Indeed, a 2011 systematic review Wachter co-authored concluded: "Mortality increases and efficiency decreases in hospitals because of year-end changeovers, although heterogeneity in the existing literature does not permit firm conclusions about the degree of risk posed"[7]. Of the six studies that had both a "good" or "very good" quality rating and a large enough sample size to detect statistically significant differences in mortality, four of them reported a mortality increase.

If we work on the basis of a reasonable possibility that hospital deaths truly do rise when new doctors start work, how should we make sense of this shocking finding? After years of expensive training and dedicated study, it is not a good feeling to contemplate that you might well, in spite of it all, be a ready-made disaster for your first batch of patients. But is it fair to lay the blame for excess changeover period deaths at the feet of the brand new doctors? In fact, the thing about changeover day is that *all* the training doctors change. Last year's debutants become Senior House Officers (SHOs) for the first time, a cohort of freshly minted registrars step up to a new level of responsibility, and even some of the consultants might have been last month's senior registrars. Doctors at each stage of training move, not just in level of responsibility, but between trusts, hospitals, specialties and departments too, often without the chance to pass on the institutional knowledge that is fundamental to getting things right. One retrospective cohort study of anaesthetics residents in Melbourne, Australia, found that the rate of undesirable events increased at the start of the academic year for all residents, regardless of their seniority, suggesting that systems factors and a lack of familiarity with local processes might be key parts of the problem.[8]

Unsurprisingly, none of the nuances discussed so far featured in a 2012 edition of the *Daily Mail* that quoted then National Medical Director for NHS England Sir Bruce Keogh in relation to a new pre-employment shadowing scheme as saying, "The intention is to end the so-called killing season"[9]. It was a startlingly unhelpful comment, sensationalising the story and legitimising a direct causal link between new doctors and patient deaths, favouring giving click bait to the *Daily Mail* rather than support to nervous new doctors. It was against this backdrop that we queued in the Education Centre on the morning of Black Wednesday, waiting to be handed our ID badges and computer passwords, which in theory were all we were lacking.

An ID badge that opens the doors you need it to and a computer password that works are undeniably essential, yet the idea that these things (combined with a medical degree and a GMC number) are all you need to feel ready couldn't be further from the truth. Any doctor who has been through the opening months of work will tell you that it often feels there is a gulf between the theory and the reality, between the title of doctor and feeling settled and safe working as one. Bridging this gap depends not on acquiring extra medical knowledge, but instead on the things that medical school did not teach us, the things that it could not teach us and the things that it taught us unintentionally along the way, which together form medicine's 'hidden curriculum'.

The term 'hidden curriculum' was coined in 1992 by Dixie J Anderson in an article elaborating her view of the educational experience as comprising the physical structures (facilities, tutors, logistics etc.), the traditional knowledge-based curriculum and the 'hidden curriculum'[10]. This elusive final part was described as "the indelible message, often nonverbal, that a person takes from an event or an experience . . . the essence, the soul, that which is remembered after the source is forgotten". Anderson went on to suggest that the hidden curriculum includes how we treat one another, how we manage uncertainty and errors and whether we can challenge the system when that is in the best interests of our patient. These aspects are some of the central themes of this book.

The hidden curriculum has more recently (and perhaps more formally) been defined as "the set of influences that function at the level of organisational structure and culture including, for example, implicit rules to survive the institution such as customs, rituals and taken for granted aspects"[11]. So, if the gap between the theory and the reality of doctoring is filled by the hidden curriculum, do we simply need to make it a bit less hidden, to bring the non-technical human elements of safe-care it relates to out into the light? Yes, we do, but that alone is not enough. We can do better than aiming just to understand the "implicit rules" of the system and how we should play by them. New doctors are inexperienced, but they are not stupid. They are motivated, kind, intelligent people who can think critically and creatively when encouraged to do so. Good doctoring often amounts to good problem solving, and the increasingly complex problems we are faced with need creative solutions. So no, we do not need to just learn about the implicit rules.

When it comes to coping with the truly demanding and complex challenges of starting work and then evolving as a new doctor, I think that the strategies, solutions and ways of thinking that can help us most are rarely found in the traditional medical sciences in which we were trained. Instead, they more often have their origins in fields such as psychology, anthropology, business and behavioural economics, a diverse range of areas that try to understand how we function as something we have been long before we were doctors – a human amongst humans. *The Bleep Test* also includes various stories based on the early years of my career and those of some colleagues, which show why it matters so much that we find ways to help new doctors get things right. This book is the product of my time as a new doctor. I hope it helps a little with yours.

LA

"Over the next seven years of medical training, we would go from bearing witness to medical dramas to becoming leading actors in them."

Paul Kalanithi, *When Breath Becomes Air*

1

DECISIONS, DECISIONS

HOW CAN NEW DOCTORS SAFELY DECIDE?

Safety First

Fast forward 12 months from my Black Wednesday. It was August 2019 and I had finished my first year of clinical practice, moving from the incredibly stretched and constantly busy District General Hospital (DGH) on the outskirts of the city to the University Hospital, which stood resplendent in the morning sunshine, its white panels gleaming, dominating the skyline like an alien spaceship that had landed and imposed itself for all to see. I passed through the revolving doors, instructed by a mechanical voice that seemed to be in charge of the spaceship to "please move forward!" and arrived for the trust induction. It was going to be an easy day. There were familiar faces from the last 12 months, urns of black coffee, free sandwiches for lunch and free biros from the BMA. I settled myself in for a day of talks on fire safety, wellbeing and information governance.

After induction was finished with, I began my new job on the fourth floor of the spaceship in the Intensive Care Unit (ICU). The patients arrived from all around, admitted via the Emergency Department downstairs, the wards upstairs or the operating theatres across the corridor. Some even came in helicopters or ambulances from other outlying hospitals, whose own ICUs could no longer manage their deteriorating conditions. Led by a hugely impressive, erudite and kind group of consultant intensivists and the registrars they were training, we began to help care for the sickest of the sick. In bed four we treated Maggie, a 65-year-old retired school teacher who had been rushed from the ward to the ICU when her body's immune response to a severe urine infection spiralled out of control, her blood pressure plummeting as she entered a state of septic shock. In bed nine a family began to gather around Claudette, arriving from France as news of her car accident rocked their world. And in the side room lay Bradley, a 32-year-old insurance broker admitted after taking all his mother's beta blockers over the course of a Saturday night, when his world seemed too much to bear.

Faced with the complexity and severity of their illnesses and injuries, one might think that ICU patients, who walk a precarious tightrope between life and death with the support of nurses, doctors and their machines, are at great risk and are therefore unsafe. In fact, the opposite is true. They may become clinically *unstable* and are certainly the sickest patients in the hospital, but they are also some of the safest. For this reason, when my cousin asked over a catch-up lunch "Isn't ICU a really scary place to work?" I was able to say that it wasn't, since I felt that given the seriousness of their conditions, the patients were as safe as they could be.

To understand this further, it is worth considering how patient safety is defined. NHS England says simply that it is "The avoidance of unintended or unexpected harm to people during the provision of healthcare"[12]. So how are patients in ICU any safer than those on a general ward? Whilst sources of harm such as drug errors, complications of medical procedures or misdiagnosis remain present, there is one key source of preventable harm that is much less likely in the critical care environment: unrecognised clinical deterioration. Critically unwell patients are very closely monitored in terms of nursing assessments, their observations and their blood tests. Taken together, these three things will flag most life-threatening changes in a patient's condition. You see changes sooner when you look more often.

By understanding that it is the frequency of monitoring in critical care that is so crucial to preventing unrecognised clinical deterioration, we can see more clearly what is required of new doctors as they try to maximise the safety of a much larger number of ward patients. We can't have observations or blood results 'on tap' on a normal ward, so we must prioritise issues and risk-assess patients by analysing the data we do have and, crucially, considering whether more information needs to be collected. Data-focused changes to treatment plans, such as catheterising unwell patients for accurate recording of urine output or taking a blood gas sample for immediate results, incrementally contribute to a clearer picture where better decisions can be made. When patients begin to deteriorate outside the safety of critical care levels of monitoring, we have to proactively look for ourselves, as often and from as many angles as we can.

It may sound straightforward to simply collect more information about an unwell patient, but in practice the volume of demands for an on-call doctor's time and attention are extreme. "You feel like you're spinning all these plates at once," one new doctor told me, echoing an analogy presented by Jerome Groopman in his bestselling book *How Doctors Think.*[13] As Groopman points out, "Actually it's harder than spinning plates because plate-spinning requires a single rotary motion and all the plates are of similar size and weight." When there are so many patients to attend to and so many tasks to do, how should we decide which patient to see or what to do first? In any busy on-call shift, the first decision we must make is what to prioritise. The next section will delve deeper into the 'volume problem' facing junior doctors, turning to psychological insights to suggest strategies to keep safety first and not drop any of the plates.

Information Overload and the Medical Filter

All doctors will be only too familiar with the feeling that there is simply too much to do, too many patients that need to be assessed and treated, too many blood tests or X-rays to look at, too many incoming bleeps with new questions and potential problems, and never enough time. One colleague recalled his experience of Black Wednesday, being pulled away from the ward where he had completed his pre-employment shadowing placement to another extremely busy ward because there were too few doctors. There he found a second-year doctor confronting her colossal list of jobs, on the brink of tears with such an impossible workload. The only senior person she could talk to about it was a passing gastroenterology registrar, who could offer little other than words of encouragement since he had his own long list of patients needing attention. This volume problem can be multiplied many times over when working on-call in the evenings, at weekends or at night, when just one doctor will be covering several wards and is unlikely to know the patients they are called to see.

Searching for answers about how to better handle such large lists of tasks, regular distractions and the resulting information overload, I read *The Organized Mind* by Daniel Levitin,[14] a Professor of Behavioural Psychology and Neuroscience in Montreal, Canada. The book explores how the human attentional system evolved in the past and functions today in the face of huge volumes of information, offering several ideas that can be applied to the overwhelming situation in which new doctors sometimes find themselves. One of them is the existence of an 'attentional filter', a psychological mechanism that marshals our limited attentional resources towards things that are either changing or important.

Upon graduating from medical school, you quickly find that close friends and family members treat you as the font of all medical wisdom, regardless of the ailment. Questions beginning "Can I just ask you about . . ." or "What do you think about . . ." inevitably crop up at a Sunday lunch or family gathering. You learn equally quickly that the correct answer to these well-intentioned questions is almost always "If you're worried, arrange to see your GP." *Almost* always. You wouldn't respond like that if your relative said they had sudden-onset, severe central crushing chest pain radiating down their left arm. By the same measure we are actually screening any and all symptoms mentioned to us, to the best of our ability, for anything potentially serious. We pass them all through our 'medical filter'.

Medical students and junior doctors develop a medical filter as they progress through training, which functions as a specialised version of the attentional filter, picking up on important signs and symptoms and focusing in on changes to a patient's clinical condition. The workings of the medical filter, which may operate in a subconscious or consciously expressed fashion, form the basis of 'clinical gestalt'. Gestalt is a German word translating as 'pattern or configuration', with the idea of 'clinical gestalt' pertaining to the acquired ability to intuitively recognise (and therefore pay appropriate attention to) certain clinical patterns. Although clinical gestalt may not always provide the diagnosis or tell us what we should do, it can still create that inner nudge, that little voice in the back of your mind saying that something does not fit the normal pattern, that something should not be allowed through the medical filter unchecked.

I was reminded of the importance of the medical filter soon after my twin brother Jo made his move to Cairo in August 2019 to teach primary school children in a large international school. He settled in well, adapting to life in the melting pot of North African and Middle Eastern culture and keeping the family WhatsApp well supplied with Instagrammable pictures of pyramids, churches and markets. He texted me with his medical questions, some neck pain here or an upset stomach there, but nothing very worrying. However, some months later my medical filter caught something.

> "My neck is so sore. I can hear a gentle crackling when I move it."
>
> My attention was suddenly gripped. Crackling upon moving his neck? Surely it couldn't be?
>
> "When you press on the tissues of your neck, does it make crackling noises?" I responded.
>
> "Yep. Exactly. It feels like bubble wrap is being popped. What does that mean? I've never had this before."
>
> "Go to hospital. Now."

As Jo hurriedly packed a bag for hospital, alarmed by my urgency, I reflected on how I had been alerted by his use of the word "crackling". I was worried that he could have subcutaneous emphysema. When he himself described it as "bubble wrap", without my suggesting the analogy, I was convinced. There was nothing else this could be. Nine hours, four doctors and one CT scan later, the hospital in Cairo was convinced too. They diagnosed a pneumomediastinum – air in the chest in the space between the two lungs. He was observed for three days, quickly being moved into a nicer side room once it was realised his international school's health insurance would pay for it, and eventually let home when no sinister cause was found. "That's the most common thing, no serious cause found, totally benign," an emergency medicine friend at Yale reassured me. "Probably due to violent coughing or something."

Nevertheless, I knew I had done the right thing. Subcutaneous emphysema is a rare sign I had seen only twice before. The second time had been only a few months previously in a post-operative patient with an un-resolved pneumothorax. Whilst waiting for a new chest drain to release the expanding collection of air that was pressing on his lung, subcutaneous emphysema had dramatically spread across his chest and neck. Alerted by a physiotherapist's comment that the patient was starting to look a little more tired, I dashed back to his room, found that his oxygen requirements had increased five-fold, and escalated his case to critical care. The patient was stabilised and left hospital a couple of weeks later, but it nevertheless cemented the significance of subcutaneous emphysema in my mind. In this way, our medical filter is primed by both the recency and saliency of clinical events, reconfiguring itself in response to our accumulation of experience. It is dynamic and constantly updating.

Although new doctors may have little or no experience of certain syndromes or diseases, raising the possibility of holes within the filter, medical school does focus heavily on things that are common and things that are life-threatening. Therefore, we do possess a filter that has been maturing over some years and has reached the stage when it can be usefully deployed. Having confidence that, whilst we still have much to learn, we are well equipped to spot problems, assess risks and prioritise our patients accordingly can reduce the stressful overload of the volume problem. The medical filter underpins our task prioritisation, and it allows the volume of work to become less intimidating once a portion of it has been safely filtered. And if our prioritisation is reliable, if we know that we *are* dealing with the most pressing issue first, we can confidently avoid an error-strewn practice when overloaded with work – multitasking.

Multitasking Muddles

Emblazoned across the back cover of *The Organized Mind* is the message: "Multitasking is a bad way to do nearly everything." The simplicity of this statement was one of the things that first drew me to the book, resonating with mistakes I knew I had been making on the wards. When I first started doing ward cover shifts, pulled this way and that between numerous different patients and jobs, I would task switch extremely frequently. When bleeped with another request to see a patient whilst mid-way through a job, I would often mistakenly believe that the new request simply couldn't wait, adding finishing off the job I was abandoning to the ever-growing list. This then required me to return at a later stage to the ward I was leaving. Although many patients do need to be re-reviewed later in a shift, too much task switching when you're in the middle of something is not efficient and should be avoided whenever possible. "Never do half a job, Luke," one emergency medicine trainee told me decisively.

I also struggled to fully focus on the clinical problem at hand when I was still half-consciously mulling over or worrying about the previous one. Levitin writes, "Multitasking is the enemy of a focused attentional system. . . . We can't truly think about or attend to all these things at once, so our brains flit from one to another, each time with a neurobiological switching cost"[15]. But how can we truly avoid multi-tasking when there are so many patients to look after, so many plates we need to keep spinning? I think there is a distinction to be made between *intentional* physical task switching and *unintentional* mental task switching. *Intentional* switching is helpful, resulting from a clear decision that the first task has been adequately dealt with, at least for now, and we can move on, with a clear plan for when (and under what circumstances or parameters) we will choose to return to it. *Unintentional* switching between problems, however, is unhelpful and distracting. Anxiously flitting between issues within the confines of our over-burdened mental storage tank can be a drain on precious cognitive resources.

In order to limit this mental self-distraction and worry, to be more mindful or more 'in the moment' with the clinical problem we're dealing with, we need to have a high degree of confidence that the task at hand is the most urgent one and that everything else can safely wait. Establishing with some certainty that these two conditions are met can facilitate a calming focus on the patient in front of us. Whilst the medical filter forms the basis for safe task prioritisation, we need to be sure that we have a grasp of all the moving parts. We need a strategy to maintain an organised medical mind.

The Paper Brain

Levitin is clear that the single most beneficial step towards an organised mind, something fundamental to our avoiding dropping the plates, "is to shift the burden of organizing from our brains to the external world"[16]. He explains that this is not a reflection of inadequate human hard-drive space, but a result of how externalising the organising process can make our memory storage and retrieval mechanisms less error-prone. The safest of new doctors will not necessarily be the ones with prize-winning firsts in medical school, but the ones with the most organised medical minds. And that probably includes carrying the neatest and most organised pieces of paper.

Aside from those junior doctors working in hospitals with a functional digital alternative (a rarity in the NHS), most rely heavily on paper lists of patients and tasks. You quickly learn to write down *everything*, realising that the volume and nature of potential distractions liable to arise at any moment means you cannot rely on remembering anything. Although not ideal from an information governance perspective due to the risk of dropping them in a public space, paper lists will remain essential until a digital solution can be adopted. This may be some time away, given that parts of the NHS are still using fax machines.

I once saw a consultant surgeon reprimand a new registrar when he saw the state of his paper list. You couldn't argue with the fact that it looked a total mess. Taking another list from the hand of a second registrar, which was beautifully organised with the patients' identity stickers in a column down the left-hand side and the relevant tasks running down the right-hand column, he brandished it as evidence saying, "When you present the patients to me, this is what I want to see!" This may seem unnecessarily pernickety and fussy. What does it matter to the consultant how the registrar writes his list? So long as he remembers everything, can't he just do it his own way? In fact, the encounter revealed the consultant's much higher levels of confidence in the second registrar who appeared to be running a tighter ship.

So how can we best utilise the humble paper list? The key insight is to not only externalise the *remembering* of content, but also to externalise the *organisation* of that content. I soon realised after a few on-call shifts that long printed lists of all the patients on the wards I was covering were of little use. Although they contained useful handover information, most of the patients on the list were not of present concern, so served only as distractors that increased the search time when trying to retrieve information for unwell patients I did need to know about. These comprehensive patient lists are good for routine ward rounds in which every patient is seen in sequence but are not usefully organised for prioritising work during a busy on-call.

Instead, I started taking blank paper like the surgical registrar, collecting identity stickers for any patient I was reviewing. Since reading *The Organized Mind*, I now divide the paper into three sections and collect the patient stickers in a particular way. Daniel Levitin recalls working as a personal assistant for a successful businessman who instructed him to sort the mail into four categories:

1. Things that need to be dealt with right away
2. Things that are important but can wait
3. Things that are not important and can wait
4. Things to be thrown out

It struck me that most clinical tasks junior doctors are bleeped to deal with can fit nicely into these categories. For example, a patient with sudden gastrointestinal bleeding and a falling blood pressure would be category 1, so her sticker goes on the first page. Page 1 is strictly reserved for acutely unwell patients. A patient with uncontrolled pain would be category 2, so his sticker goes on the next page. Pain is unpleasant and may have a serious cause but cannot kill you in and of itself. A request for a cannula would depend on which IV medicines it was needed for – it could be category 2 or category 3. And the bleeps such as prescribing paracetamol or laxatives can be dealt with and then thrown out (category 4), which don't need their own section on the paper since you're not even keeping a sticker.

With the accumulation of experience, operating this kind of triage system becomes easier and more automatic. You learn to phone the ward in question and gather pertinent information from the nurses. Finding out whether Margaret who has had a fall on the ward has hit her head or is taking any blood thinners will help decide which category she fits into. And taking a few extra moments to establish that Bert who has returned from theatre with a blood pressure of 90/60 mmHg is in fact awake, talking, passing urine via his catheter, not reporting any symptoms and has an epidural in situ that likely explains his relative hypotension is reassuring and helps to sort him into category 2 rather than category 1. The word 'triage' comes from the French verb 'trier' meaning 'to sort'. The value of proactively trying to sort tasks by fact finding and listening to the nurse's concerns cannot be overstated.

Whilst I have designated category 1 tasks as 'things that need to be dealt with right away', there is in fact a higher category, a set of situations that must bypass this organisational structure entirely. Crucially, they are 'things that need to be dealt with *now*, and not by us alone'. Sooner or later, we will find a patient who is so dangerously unwell that the first decision you take must be to call the medical emergency team to attend. This is the question of deciding when a patient is peri-arrest and calling the cavalry.

ABCDE and Calling the Cavalry

It is usually expected that new doctors will review patients' case notes, take a medical history, perform a clinical examination and order any suitable tests before diagnosing and treating the condition as far as they are able. This is the traditional approach to clinical medicine: history, examination, investigations, diagnosis and treatment. However, when faced with an acutely unwell or deteriorating patient, it is not the correct order of doing things and overly conscientious adherence to this usual structure will result in delays to urgent patient management. Instead, we are taught to do a systematic ABCDE assessment of the patient's airway, breathing, circulation, disability and exposure. This alternative method enables rapid identification and treatment of potentially life-threatening issues that need to be immediately addressed.

Whilst the vast majority of situations can be dealt with, at least initially, via the traditional medical work-up or an ABCDE assessment from the junior doctor, there is a need to recognise a patient who is in such an extreme situation that trying to manage by yourself will put you so far out of your depth that it is essential to call some experienced team members to come running *before* you do anything else. This option to urgently call the crash team for a peri-arrest patient can be taken immediately upon meeting a patient, during the ABCDE assessment upon identifying a serious problem, or later if a patient is rapidly deteriorating despite the current treatment plan.

In her bestselling book *Your Life in My Hands*, Rachel Clarke recounts how, on her first-ever night shift, she was called to see an extremely sick man suffering from acute heart failure but was not bleeped back by her registrar when she phoned for help.[17] She left the patient's bedside to fetch a senior doctor, during which time the patient arrested, going on to require defibrillation, resuscitation and transfer to the ICU. Dr Clarke reflected that

> I lacked the practical knowledge that a crash call is appropriate for anyone you think is about to fall off a cliff, not only those who have already done so. Perhaps it is the fear of being seen to do the wrong thing – the embarrassment of mistaking a patient's minor unwellness for a full-blown emergency – that holds young doctors back from calling the cavalry. This reticence has the potential to cost patients their lives.

So, how do we know when a patient is peri-arrest? When I began working as a new doctor, I had assumed that I would know easily enough when to 'hit the twos', dialling the 2222 number that is now used across the UK for a crash call. I had done six years of medical school, undertaken elective modules in anaesthetics and resuscitation, and seen some desperately sick patients along the way. "I know a dangerously unwell person when I see one," I reassured myself. I was confident enough in my 'end-of-bed-ogram', which is a good word for simply standing at the foot of the patient's bed and guesstimating where they are on a scale ranging from totally fine to near-death. This crude but reasonably effective method relies on pattern recognition, subconsciously and rapidly relating the present cues to prior knowledge and experience using what Daniel Kahneman defines in *Thinking, Fast and Slow* as 'System 1' thinking.[18] Our evolutionarily wired ability to 'Think Fast' and recognise impending danger much faster than we can explicitly say how or why we know this danger to be there may allow us to call 2222 with the stethoscope still around our necks, without even touching the patient. If we do not rapidly reach a judgement via System 1 thinking, we then attempt to reach our decision with a slower, explicit process of deductive reasoning – this is Kahneman's System 2 or 'Thinking Slow'.

My first job as a new doctor was a four-month rotation in orthogeriatrics, which is a fancy word meaning 'elderly care medicine for neck of femur fracture patients'. A short time into this placement I was called over by one of the nurses to "just have a look" at Gerald, an elderly man in Bed 6. Arriving at the bed space, I clocked his observations chart, which was not at all reassuring, and thought that Gerald was failing the end-of-bed-ogram by some margin. His eyes were closed, his skin was sweaty and clammy, and his rapid shallow breathing filled me with dread.

I mentally ticked off A for airway but was stuck considering the obvious issue with B for breathing. I was trying to join the dots but knew nothing about Gerald's medical history or problems this admission, was scrambling around for answers and beginning to arrive at the conclusion that we needed help. However, before I could communicate this to anyone, I heard Sally our ward clerk say matter-of-factly from behind the desk "Oh I don't like the look of him, I'm putting out the twos!" And so, the crash team was called. They diagnosed him with a severe chest infection and exacerbation of heart failure, optimised his medical treatment and, after discussions with his family, put in place a DNACPR form. Gerald died the following day.

At the time I felt ashamed and wondered what the ward staff must have thought. What use was I as a doctor if it had required our ward clerk, with no medical training, to intervene and make the correct decision? But I shouldn't have been, for this is the speed of System 1 thinking. Through her accumulated observations across hundreds of shifts on the ward, Sally had built up a mental picture of the critically unwell elderly patient and had acted accordingly. With my more limited experience, I had been deploying System 2 thinking, trying to make sense of the signs in front of me in the context of an unknown clinical history, which was much, much slower.

The fact that new doctors often lack the depth of experience required to reliably pattern recognise with System 1 is a problem that we will explore further. For now, the lesson is that if you, *or anyone else working on the ward*, have the gut feeling that it's time to call the cavalry, then just do it. Where the patient appears to have current or impending failure of any one of A, B, C or D, that is not fixable with the knowledge, equipment or skillset to hand, calling for help is a necessity. Even if you are wrong and the patient is not in fact life-threateningly unwell, the mild embarrassment will fade quickly, and you can be sure that the senior doctors attending on the crash team will have forgotten the whole thing by teatime. This is infinitely preferable to the alternative possibility of missing the boat and failing to call for help, an outcome that would prove troubling and deeply guilt provoking for the doctor, but potentially catastrophic for the patient. Having the humility to ask for help at an early stage is a key skill for new doctors, but the situation is not always as dramatic as a peri-arrest patient. In routine, everyday practice, we need to know when we don't know.

The Art of Not Knowing

"I don't know. I don't know. Say it again and again until you get used to saying it!" Professor Ashok Handa ordered the rows of students filling the John Radcliffe Hospital lecture theatre. We weren't sure what was coming next, but my group was situated far enough up the steep banked seating that we felt unlikely to be singled out for questioning. "It's something you lot find hard to say, because you're all bright and intelligent people, but you need to get good at saying it. I don't know! I don't know!" The lecture about general surgery continued and our seating strategy proved pointless as Prof Handa rotated the question answering around the room, demanding at any point when an answer was not forthcoming that the question be passed on to an adjacent colleague. Nothing indecisive was accepted. "No, don't guess. If you don't know, that's fine, it's why you're here, but say it – I don't know."

With the benefit of hindsight, we were not only being taught about the anatomical difference between the midpoint of the inguinal ligament and the mid-inguinal point, or about direct and indirect hernias, or about any of the surgical topics we needed to understand for the upcoming final exams. The broader objective was to get us to recognise and accept our knowledge gaps, and to respond accordingly, passing the question on to someone a few chairs along who might have the answer. In a room full of students where an unhealthy combination of exam anxiety and perfectionist tendencies was pretty much the norm, accepting that we did not know could be a difficult conclusion to arrive at. Yet it was a training exercise for what was to come. It sometimes surprises patients and their families that somebody who has been in medical school for six years, passed numerous examinations and has 'Doctor' in front of their name will so frequently not know what to do, but the truth is that it is very common. In these situations, just like in the lecture theatre, we are required quite reasonably not to guess and to pass the question to a colleague. But is practising safely in the early years really this simple? What is the reality for new doctors when faced with these decisions?

Decision Escalation, a.k.a. 'Bumping Up the Chain'

Following on from our initiation in the art of admitting "I don't know", it was reiterated to us as graduating medical students that when uncertain we should always seek advice from a senior colleague, something I refer to as 'bumping decisions up the chain'. The formal term for this is 'escalation'. Each doctor can escalate the problem to a more senior clinician. When consultants are unsure, they may seek help from a colleague within their own specialty or ask for advice from another specialty. As a system of working, it makes obvious sense and is essential for keeping patients safe. GMC guidance requires doctors to "recognise and work within the limits of [their] competence"[19]. Underlining that new doctors are not expected to deal with everything independently is also intended to be reassuring, highlighting that support should be available when required. It reminded me of Albus Dumbledore's famous assertion, "help will always be given at Hogwarts to those who ask for it"[20].

But hospital is not Hogwarts and there may be barriers to decision escalation working as intended. Firstly, the immediate senior decision maker may be unresponsive or unable to review the patient, leading to delays whilst alternative help is sought. A second, often related, problem is that the rate of escalation within and between hospital teams may be outstripped by the pace of change in a patient's condition, meaning that critical decisions or actions are not delivered within the required timeframe. These issues are exacerbated in an understaffed and over-stretched system, but they can be partly mitigated if we have considered in advance the likely timings for obtaining help, have a low threshold for seeking it elsewhere and know how to do so. However, there remains a single, more fundamental flaw in the chain of escalation – what if we don't know that we don't know?

Insight Failure

Crucially, decision escalation relies on each doctor having enough insight into his or her own understanding of a clinical problem to correctly pass a decision up the chain. It is an over-simplification to assume that "everything will be fine because, if you don't know, just ask". Bumping something up the chain still requires us to decide that we are not competent to decide, and this decision is subject to the full range of human cognitive biases just like any other. In other words, a decision cannot be avoided. Whether you decide to act or decide to bump the issue up the chain, you still have to choose. Getting this choice wrong represents an insight failure.

The only way to eliminate this possibility entirely would be to discuss *everything* with a senior doctor, i.e., not to make any decisions independently. In environments where every patient will get a senior review, such as clerking in the Acute Medical Unit (AMU) or the Surgical Assessment Unit (SAU), this strategy is perhaps tenable. New doctors can see a patient and present a proposed management plan to a senior colleague who will then either give it the go ahead or make alterations and additions, often checking or clarifying some elements of the history and clinical examination themselves. The new doctor can then safely learn from any changes. This is probably what was envisioned by the GMC in its *Outcomes for provisionally registered doctors* document, highlighting the aims for first-year doctors to be "using medicines safely and effectively (under supervision)" and to be "managing acutely ill patients under supervision"[21]. The only insight required of new doctors in this setting is to establish that no time-critical decisions beyond their abilities are needed prior to the planned senior review. If they are, experienced senior nurses have usually noticed this already. In general, the management decisions here are automatically bumped.

Unfortunately, the reality is that new doctors are widely required to practise at weekends, in the evening or at night, in ward cover roles that do not have this in-built safety net of an automatic senior review.

Here, the help will *only* be given to those who ask for it. Further, discussing every decision with a senior colleague cannot continue indefinitely, otherwise the can is simply kicked down the road and we will never progress. Regardless of how teams and systems are structured, there remains a necessity to learn to decide if we can decide, and to face the associated risk of insight failure.

Having perfect insight into one's own abilities could be described as demonstrating a perfect linear relationship between competence and confidence. Decisions and tasks firmly within your grasp would be efficiently managed without undue fear or anxiety, whilst those beyond your limits would be recognised as such, with low confidence of success triggering an escalation up the chain. However, psychological research by Dunning and Kruger in 1999 revealed that the relationship between competence and confidence is anything but linear.[22] They showed that those with the lowest competence had some of the highest levels of confidence in their own abilities, a situation widely described as 'the peak of Mount Stupid'. This stage was then followed by a sharp and sustained drop in confidence as competence increased, followed eventually by a more linear rise in confidence associated with the development of true expertise or mastery (Figure 1.1). The effect is best explained by the fact that, when we are truly ignorant, we have so little knowledge or understanding of the problem or task that we *think* it is straightforward. Ignorance may be bliss, but the Dunning–Kruger effect shows that it is also blind.

Professor David Matthews, one of my former tutors at Harris Manchester College, was aware of the importance of insight in managing clinical uncertainty, so had an interesting curveball he would use when interviewing potential medical students.

> At least once in every interview, I follow up a candidate's response by asking 'In percentage terms, how sure are you about that?' If they're correct and confident about it, that's fine, and if they're wrong and appropriately uncertain that's also fine. It's more worrying if they're very wrong but very certain that they're right.

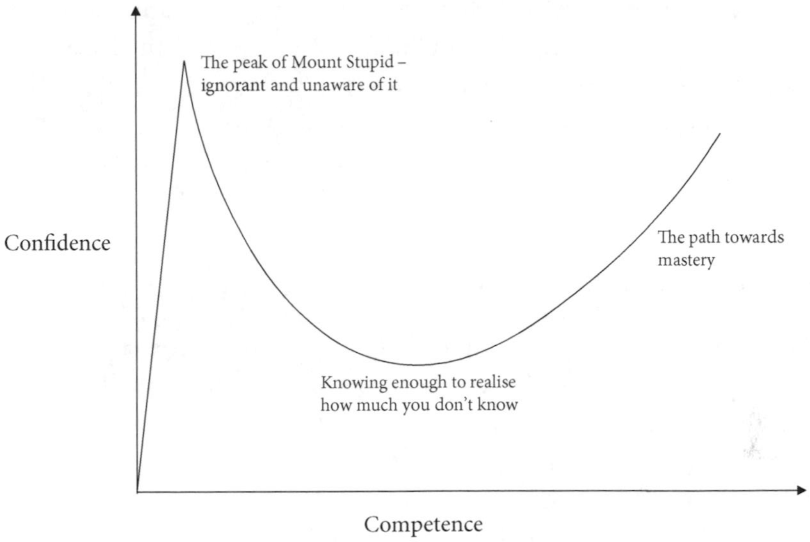

Figure 1.1 Ignorance is blind – The Dunning–Kruger effect. (After Dunning and Kruger, 1999.)

Rather than simply being an instrument to assess whether the candidates are well-adjusted young people, this line of questioning acknowledges the Dunning–Kruger effect to screen for potential doctors who have so completely missed the point of the topic or its complexity that they display no insight into their mistakes.

If the Dunning–Kruger effect is hard-wired into human psychology, can anything be done about it? Can we better recognise when we are sitting atop Mount Stupid and straying into a blind spot? The accumulation of theoretical knowledge and practical skills at medical school should in theory shift students towards the middle of the Dunning–Kruger curve, moving future doctors away from the dangerous far left-hand side. An ideal outcome may be where new doctors are understandably inexpert in many areas, but have become experienced enough to recognise the issues at hand and will therefore be appropriately lacking in confidence to try and manage everything by themselves. However, the somewhat random nature of experiential learning during clinical training, combined with the fact that no medical school curriculum in the world can adequately teach and examine the full breadth of modern medicine, means that blind spots are inevitable. The problem remains – can we see where we are blind?

Seeing in Blindness – Knowing What We Don't Know

To illustrate the problem of blind spot bias we can borrow and adapt a technique from cognitive psychology called the 'Johari Window'[23]. In 1955, the psychologists Joseph Luft (Jo) and Harrington Ingham (Hari) asked participants in a self-help group to select adjectives that they felt applied to their own personalities, and then to select adjectives that they felt described their peers. These various traits could then be organised into a four-squared grid according to whether the participant, their peers, both parties or neither had picked them. Adjectives that both parties selected fell into the 'Arena', traits self-selected by the individual but not by the peers were classed as 'Façade', whereas characteristics recognised by the peers but not by the individual represented the 'Blind Spot'. The fourth quadrant, 'The Unknown', contained the adjectives nobody had selected, either because they truly did not apply to the person or because neither party had recognised that they did.

As we consider various strands of clinical information in pursuit of a decision, the framework of the Johari Window reminds us that we are not sole actors. Our appreciation of a patient's problem and what *we* deem relevant information constitutes only one perspective, one angle and one data set, which cannot paint the whole picture. Our information will overlap only partially with the data known to others such as a nurse, physiotherapist, family member or the patient themselves. In his book *Rebel Ideas: The Power of Diverse Thinking*, sports journalist, author and performance consultant Matthew Syed argues that considering truly diverse viewpoints can produce innumerable benefits across a range of sectors from counterterrorism to business to healthcare.[24] He recalls the work of Katherine Phillips from Columbia Business School, who demonstrated the power of adding a non-white team member to a pair of white individuals in a study that gave different groups of participants murder mystery style puzzles to solve.[25] The more racially diverse teams with a so-called outsider's perspective to draw on were successful in solving the mystery 75% of the time, compared to only 54% in the homogeneous white groups. Dealing with undifferentiated medical problems is often said to be detective work, so these murder mystery puzzle findings may be more applicable to medicine than it would appear!

Blind spot information that is known to others, but not to the decision-maker, represents a serious missed opportunity to mitigate Dunning–Kruger bias. Equally, unshared information held by the decision-maker alone risks misunderstandings and miscommunications further down the line and could have prompted other helpful input from team members had it been shared. The truly useful and actionable information lies in the 'Arena', where it is shared and understood by all clinicians and their patient, forming the building blocks for what is widely referred to in the patient safety and human factors literature as a 'shared mental model'. With everyone singing from the same hymn sheet, better decisions become more likely.

At the point of decision-making, reframing the Johari Window (Figure 1.2) shows that we can expand the team's Arena. We can reduce our personal blind spot by appreciating that it is only a proportion of the unknown information that is truly unknown to everybody – more is within our grasp if we proactively ask for the perspectives and feedback of others. Equally, we can lessen our façade, sharing our information by voicing our thoughts and concerns to those around us. This could be anything from the most junior doctor finding the courage to say that they heard a soft heart murmur in a septic patient when

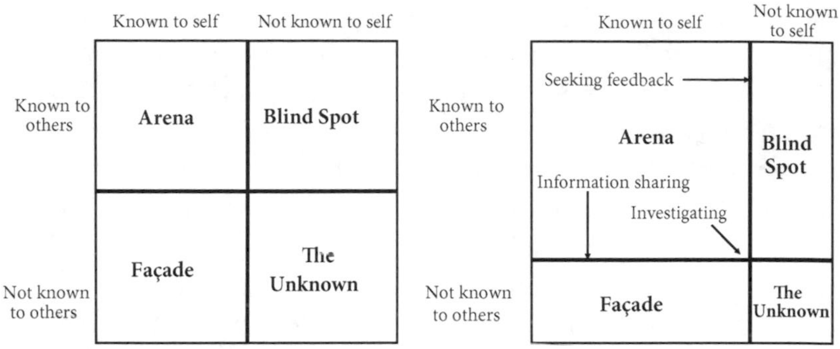

Figure 1.2 Reframing the Johari Window. (After Luft and Ingham, 1955.)

nobody else remembered to listen, raising the possibility of infectious endocarditis, or admitting to the team that Mr Jacobsen's INR is probably still high because his Warfarin had not been paused as instructed. Finally, if the decision can safely be delayed, we may choose to order further investigations, attempting to push back the frontiers of the truly unknown information.

Junior doctors are presented with clinical problems encompassing everything from "Will you prescribe some paracetamol for Mrs North?" (almost always yes), through to horrifyingly unwell patients who require urgent senior input, and everything in between. So how much information need be in the Arena before we can safely decide? When we have appropriately investigated a problem, shared our knowledge with the team, listened to their perspectives and insights and been aware of and done our utmost to avoid an insight failure, we find that we have come full circle. We must decide. Do we act ourselves or bump the problem up the chain? How certain should we be?

One colleague described his approach like this: "I ask myself what is the worst thing this could possibly be? How likely are the various possibilities? With this in mind, how comfortable will I be with my name on paper next to this decision?" Unless we are feeling very comfortable, it's time to bump the decision and ask for help. Although we might wish we had known what to do or feel that we *should* have known what to do, a timely acceptance that we need help is not a weakness but a great strength. Medicine is not straightforward. It is supposed to be difficult. "There is zero shame in calling for help," my flatmate Dan, an SHO in general surgery, reassured me.

Indeed, even for the consultants whose expertise and experience can hugely expand the Arena on a problem, the reality of our imperfect science means that the unknown portion of the window is always present to some degree. In his book *Critical*, ICU consultant Matt Morgan makes the case that "I do not know" are the four "most under-used words in medicine", explaining, "People want plans, they want certainty, they want answers gained from years of education and experience. And doctors want to give this. Admitting to yourself that uncertainty cannot be eliminated takes guts"[26]. At the start of our careers, there is a tendency to think that the uncertainty we are currently wrestling with will go away with time, if only we could hurry up and become registrars or consultants. Unfortunately, this is a pipe dream. New consultants in their mid-30s can often be heard commenting on how much simpler things seemed back when they were a registrar. Uncertainties will change and will evolve in content and nature as we progress, but doubts will remain however senior we become. The art of not knowing is something we have to learn and become comfortable with.

Know Thy Enemy, Know Thy Self

The proverb "if you know your enemies and know yourself, you will not be imperilled in a hundred battles" is attributed to the Chinese general Sun Tzu (circa. 6000 BC) in his treatise on military strategy *The Art of War*.[27] Away from the battlefields of Ancient China, the idea of seeking to understand 'enemy' and 'self' can equally be applied to seeking to understand a clinical problem (the enemy) and ourselves as the problem solver (self) when we are trying to make safe decisions. Knowing the problem is the simpler bit – we either learnt enough about it in medical school, or we can get help from a textbook, guideline or colleague, providing that we look for it. Knowing ourselves is harder and requires detailed reflection on both how we approach decision-making and how our approaches can be derailed by human cognitive biases, leading to faulty reasoning and bad decisions. So how do junior doctors go about making clinical decisions?

In 2015, a trainee GP called Emily Adams led a qualitative research study investigating clinical reasoning of junior doctors in emergency medicine (EM), a specialty which, the authors pointed out, represents a "demanding clinical reasoning domain, especially for junior doctors who lack experience"[28]. Adams was joined on the research team by Lois Brand, one of my former tutors and an experienced EM consultant and educationalist at the University of Oxford, and Carl Heneghan, who is a practising GP and director of Oxford's Centre for Evidence-Based Medicine. The team conducted a combination of interviews and focus groups involving a total of 37 junior doctors ranging from between two- and four-years post-qualification. The recordings from these sessions were then analysed and coded to draw out emerging themes that could be developed into a working model of the juniors' predominant clinical reasoning strategies. A schematic version is shown in Figure 1.3. The model works from an acceptance of Kahneman's dual cognition theory (DCT) of two systems: fast intuitive pattern recognition (System 1) and slow, deliberate

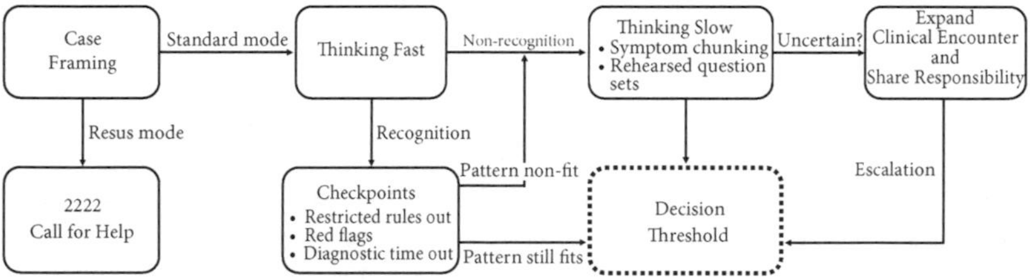

Figure 1.3 Emergency medicine junior doctors' clinical reasoning model. (After Adams and colleagues, 2017.)

hypothetico-deductive reasoning (System 2) as being broadly applicable to clinical decision-making.

This model revolves around three sequential phases of clinical reasoning. Firstly, juniors engaged in 'case framing', combining a review of triage notes, referral letters and online clinic letters with 'the eyeball test' or 'end-of-bed-ogram', which is a System 1 (thinking fast) process. Although the eyeball test is rapid and intuitive, it was revealed to be based on sound consideration of clinical features such as level of consciousness, hydration status and skin colour that the juniors explicitly verbalised as relevant factors when questioned. In the second phase of 'evolving reasoning', the juniors either pursued a diagnosis based on early System 1 recognition of a key feature or collections of features or responded to non-recognition by switching to hypothetico-deduction with methods such as 'symptom chunking' (separately analysing each presenting symptom) or using rehearsed question sets. Early pattern recognition in this phase was followed up with checkpoints such as checking for red flag features of a particular complaint. If any checkpoint strategies challenged the working diagnosis, leading to a situation of pattern non-fit, the juniors instituted hypothetico-deductive reasoning (thinking slow) as they would have done with an initial reaction of non-recognition. If a decision-making threshold was still not reached, phase three of 'ongoing uncertainty' involved expanding the clinical encounter to allow more time for test results to be returned, the situation to develop, reassessment or re-clerking based on new thoughts, or escalating to a senior to share the responsibility for decision-making. Each of these responses to ongoing uncertainty would expand the Arena portion of Johari's window.

Although the most junior doctors included in the study were second-year doctors and it focused exclusively on decision-making in the Emergency Department, the three phases of clinical reasoning are also applicable to the situation of new doctors confronting decisions on the wards. In the same way that the EM juniors used case framing to initially decide whether a patient could be assessed in the standard way or needed an ABCDE approach and/or transfer to the resuscitation room, the first decision point for new doctors when reviewing a sick ward patient is always "to 2222 or not to 2222". Once happy that a crash call is not currently necessary, they can proceed to decide whether a traditional medical approach or an ABCDE evaluation is more appropriate. Accurately case framing ward patients in this way and reflecting that thought process in the style of documentation conveys that the relative severity of the situation has been considered. I find it strange when a clinical examination is documented as an ABCDE assessment even when the problem is minor or trivial. I prefer to reserve this style of documentation for patients who are unwell or deteriorating, signalling as much to myself as to others that I am thinking in 'resuscitation mode'. Phases two and three of the clinical reasoning model are also easily applicable to ward-based medicine.

Regardless of the clinical context in which the patient is seen, there are some universal considerations arising from the model proposed by Adams and colleagues and the application of DCT to junior doctors' clinical reasoning that are worth exploring further. The first point is that System 1-based diagnosis according to pattern recognition happens more often than we should probably be comfortable with. Because the classic, easily recognisable presentations of diseases taught and examined in medical school occur much less frequently in real-life Emergency Departments or hospital wards than they do in the textbooks, early-career doctors may sometimes lack the extensively developed mental bank of clinical experience required to safely deploy System 1-type thinking. The hectic wards and departments, queues of unwell patients on trolleys, 4-hour waiting time targets and relentless bleeps charitably described by Adams and colleagues as "contextual demands" push juniors towards the mental "heuristics" associated with System 1 thinking, but it is known that these shortcuts are less likely to have been reliably developed in more junior clinicians.[29] Attempting to think fast and take mental shortcuts exposes us to a large range of possible cognitive errors that can lead to mistakes being made.

The number and variety of possible errors is staggering, but a very readable and comprehensive summary compiled by Justin Morgenstern is available on his "First10EM" blog.[30] Jerome Groopman in *How Doctors Think* draws our attention to the '3As of thinking traps': anchoring (fixating on one possible diagnosis and failing to adequately consider alternatives), availability bias (over-estimating the likelihood of a diagnosis simply because similar cases have been seen recently) and attribution error (over-weighting the importance of personality-based judgements of a patient's presentation, such as attributing a low GCS in a homeless man to drunkenness and failing to diagnose sepsis).[31] The concept of 'triage cueing', in which the clinical area where a patient is seen biases the diagnosis, is also concerning and suggests that geography can become destiny. One participant in Adams' research recalled seeing a 26-year-old patient who had come into ED minors reporting some black stool and he had said, "Okay, yes, yes, that's fine", when in fact the patient was suffering a major gastrointestinal haemorrhage. When it comes to clinical metacognition, which is thinking about how we think clinically, it really matters that we are up to speed on cognitive errors. Groopman comments, "Of course, a doctor must know physiology and pathology and pharmacology. But he should also be schooled in heuristics – in the power and necessity of shortcuts, and in their pitfalls and dangers".[32]

Another consideration from all this thinking about thinking is the question of whether we can be the masters of our own System 1 and System 2 – can we decide when to think fast and when to think slow? Adams and colleagues state "intuitive and analytical cognition are in constant dialectic in all three phases [of clinical reasoning]", suggesting that our thought process naturally swings between the systems after an initial intuitive judgement is produced. But can we control how much heed we pay to each system when forming a final judgement? One piece of this puzzle is clinician-perceived complexity of the clinical problem, which is of course subject to Dunning–Kruger bias. In 2008, Mamede and colleagues found that medical residents showed significantly higher diagnostic accuracy and a switch to slower, analytical reasoning in an experimental condition where a perception of complexity was induced by telling the residents that other physicians had failed to get the diagnosis.[33] The implication of this finding is that Dunning–Kruger blind spot bias in junior doctors who have a perception of low complexity could keep them away from System 2 analytical reasoning.

It is also important to acknowledge that our cognitive response to a given scenario may well be influenced by external, situational factors not directly related to that patient's case. Our ability to make good judgements will be altered by environmental stress levels, distractions, fatigue and our current level of information overload. Given the usual volume and complexity of sick patients in our severely over-stretched health systems, how can we make better decisions under pressure?

The Cognitive Pressure Cooker – Deciding When the Heat Is On

A well-known principle in cognitive psychology is the 'stress-performance' curve, which suggests that the relationship between one's stress levels and their performance takes the form of a bell-shaped curve (Figure 1.4). Too little stress and we are inadequately stimulated

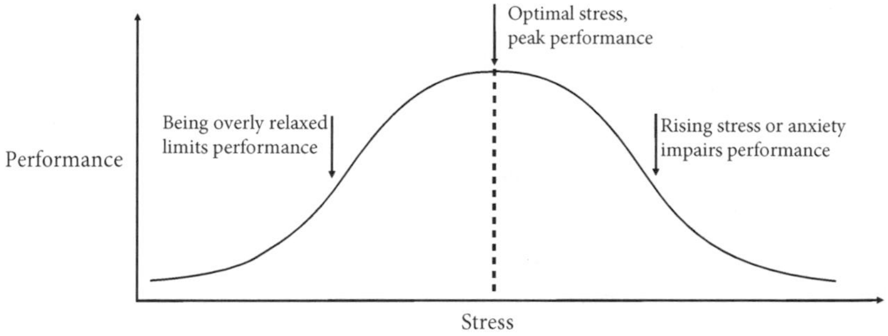

Figure 1.4 The Yerkes–Dodson (Stress-Performance) Curve. (After Yerkes and Dodson, 1908.)

to perform at our best. Too much and we become overloaded, panicked and unable to usefully deploy our skills. It seems that there is a Goldilocks zone where our stress levels can be just right. Another name for this phenomenon is the 'Yerkes–Dodson' curve, named after the scientists who developed the theory by adjusting the stress (in the form of electric shocks) applied to mice completing a maze task.[34]

In his book *Peak Performance under Pressure: Lessons from a Helicopter Rescue Doctor*, emergency medicine consultant Stephen Hearns suggests that there are three key contributing factors to the position we find ourselves in on the Yerkes–Dodson curve: our physiological stress response, information overload and, most interestingly, a phenomenon called 'cognitive appraisal'[35]. Cognitive appraisal is, Hearns explains, "how we perceive the magnitude of the situation, the risks involved and our personal ability to overcome them"[36]. If we perceive that attempting to address a problem will be extremely risky for either the patient or for ourselves, and that our problem-solving resources are likely to be overwhelmed, we are pushed to the right on the stress-performance curve.

Early on in my Intensive Care job onboard the University Spaceship, I experienced a mixture of all three elements Hearns refers to that caused me to freeze at just the wrong moment. Near the end of the day, a nurse calmly approached me at the desk and asked if I was free. I said that I was and assumed from her manner that this would be a menial prescription to write or suchlike. Saying nothing else she led me into a side room to the patient she was caring for. Still, she said nothing. I was puzzled. Still saying nothing, she jabbed her finger in the air towards her patient's monitoring screen, which I couldn't see because it was angled towards the other side of the room. I craned my head around – and stopped. The patient's systolic blood pressure was only 40 mmHg.

I froze. The way the nurse had responded to this peri-arrest situation by calmly fetching the most junior doctor on the entire ICU was so bizarre, so out of kilter with what the scenario demanded, that I was mentally thrown. Despite having completed the first year since graduating, I was truly back to square one when it came to assessing an intubated, critically unwell patient. I was not primed for such a situation, and the sudden and unexpected change of cognitive pace created such a massive physiological stress response that I entered the state of freezing, rather than even fight (beginning resuscitation) or flight (rapidly fetching help). In my head I wanted to ask for the patient to be tilted into a Trendelenburg position right away, to increase the venous return to the heart, but my lips wouldn't say the words. Luckily, before I had time to snap out of it, a Senior Sister assumed control and pulled the crash buzzer. The team arrived and rapidly diagnosed the problem, which turned out to be a kink in the line supplying noradrenaline to the patient. Once the noradrenaline was flowing properly, the blood pressure was soon corrected.

My inexperience had meant that my cognitive appraisal of the scenario was different to that of the more senior doctors. As we progress in our training and build a mental bank of similar scenarios, even the most dramatic changes in a patient's condition, such as severe desaturation or acute hypotension, begin to become more routine. They become perceived as less threatening, enabling the treating doctor to calmly achieve cognitive flow and address the issue. That's not to say it becomes easy. It is simply that with further experience, a greater proportion of the thinking can be offloaded to our intuitive, automatic System 1. Implicit, almost procedural recall of key points, algorithm steps and drug doses for use in peri-arrest scenarios comes to the fore. Understanding the type of cognitive processing we are likely to be relying on in various situations and at different stages of our progression is paramount not only for junior doctors, but also for the seniors who must supervise and train us.

Facing the Music

In this chapter we have found that the Dunning–Kruger effect, that curious non-linear relationship between self-perceived ability and actual competence, is a key cognitive bias for new doctors to understand in the early years of practice. If left unchecked, this 'blind spot bias' can worsen our decisions and reduce patient safety, and it is just one of many cognitive errors we are all vulnerable to. When stressed, overloaded and pushed for time we are more likely to attempt to take mental shortcuts and rely on quick heuristics, exposing ourselves to a wide array of cognitive bear traps to fall into. As we understand more about how junior doctors think, we can see that slow, structured and systematic reasoning is essential for new doctors as they begin to make decisions. As the US Navy SEAL saying goes, "Slow is smooth, smooth is fast."

New doctors need no reminding that their decisions, including whether to bump something up the chain, will have consequences. Although we are some years away from being 'Senior Decision Makers' (registrars or consultants), the necessity to constantly decide when to act independently and when to bump problems up the chain is inescapable. We are all clinical decision makers. This degree of responsibility for our patients, even as a junior member of the team, is fundamentally all that separates the final year medical student from the new doctor. When we wake up on Black Wednesday we have no new knowledge or skills, only the privilege of being called Doctor and the accompanying responsibility. It is the Peter Parker principle.

As we begin to accept this responsibility we see the results of our decisions, so Chapter 2 and Chapter 3 explore what it means to get things wrong and right, respectively. How should we process our failures and successes? The Canadian physician Sir William Osler, widely regarded as the father of modern medicine, titled his famous 1912 essay *Aequanimitas*,[37] which translates as 'imperturbability'. The ability to sail on an even keel and remain unperturbed seems like a useful trait, but can we really treat our triumphs and disasters just the same?

"Failure has taught me lessons I would never otherwise have understood. I have evolved more as a result of things going wrong than when everything seemed to be going right. Out of crisis has come clarity, and sometimes even catharsis."

Elizabeth Day, *How to Fail*

"Every intern makes mistakes. The important thing is neither to make the same mistakes twice nor to make a whole bunch of mistakes all at once."

Samuel Shem, *The House of God*

2

ACCIDENTAL EMERGENCIES

HOW SHOULD WE LEARN FROM OUR MISTAKES?

The Mistakes in Waiting

As the days after Black Wednesday turned into weeks and then months, I gradually became more familiar with being a new doctor. I completed the four months in orthogeriatrics with the elderly hip fracture patients and moved to a smaller hospital for the second rotation of the year, this time in general medicine. The Small Hospital was a kinder place to work than the District General Hospital. Charity volunteers waved good morning and the consultants knew your name. The registrar I was paired with for on-call shifts was competent and kind, and I felt that with her to turn to for help things would be ok. I began to enjoy going to work for the first time, Christmas was coming and what was more, the Rota Gods had been in my favour – I was not on call until the 28th of December, so could combine some annual leave with the bank holidays to have a proper break. I knew that in future years I would not be so fortunate as to spend Christmas with family, but for now . . . well that was next year's problem. I booked a train for the 22nd and, grateful for the six days off, packed some things to head home.

In an effort to work up an appetite for eating too much at various Christmas parties, I arranged to play squash with Tom, who had been our babysitter when we were small. We had always pushed our luck with bedtime on those Saturday nights, demanding to stay up and watch *Who Wants to Be a Millionaire?* Tom had responded with a compromise, ruling that we could stay up . . . until we got a question wrong. Lifelines were not permitted, and final answers were required before the contestant selected theirs. He correctly banked on the difficulty ramping up beyond the £8000 mark and almost always got us packed off to sleep less than 30 minutes late. I smiled at the memory. It was hard to believe that was 15 years ago.

"How are you doing? How have things been so far?" Tom asked. "Have you made any mistakes yet? You must have done." I paused. This was much more interesting, and more confronting, than the usual predictable questions about whether I was enjoying it and whether I knew what I was going to specialise in. Occasionally, when catching up with non-medical friends there is somebody who wants to know what it is really like. No, what it is *really* like, to start working as a new doctor.

I could tell that Tom was in this category, so recounted some of my early errors: prescribing a patient's anti-hypertensives for the woman in the adjacent bed who shared her initials, forgetting to check some last-minute blood tests for a patient being discharged and not prioritising looking at a "lump" that turned out to be an expanding haematoma. "Luckily the patients were ok," I recalled. "But sooner or later there will be a time when something goes wrong and the patient isn't ok, won't there?" Tom responded. "With the working conditions in the NHS it's inevitable, isn't it? But it won't be your fault, because you won't have meant to get it wrong, you won't have done it on purpose." I wasn't so sure. I was pretty certain I would still feel completely responsible.

Despite having no medical training whatsoever, Tom's words were relevant and wise, and with the benefit of hindsight they were prescient. Although I knew that he was right and further mistakes would occur at some point, my mistakes in waiting turned out to be closer than I thought. However, I wanted to believe that these errors, if truly inevitable, would not lead to patients being harmed. Surely there could be a way to move safely up the learning curve.

Safely up the Learning Curve

In his book *Black Box Thinking*, Matthew Syed argues that the value of practice lies in its ability to provide a steady stream of mistakes from which we can learn.[38] "It is better to fail in practice . . . than on the big stage itself," he writes. "The more we can fail in practice, the more we can learn, enabling us to succeed when it really matters." These ideas are intuitive and convincing, but sit far more comfortably in the context of table tennis (my own and Syed's former sport) than in healthcare delivery, the subject of much of *Black Box Thinking*. If, as Syed puts it, success "is built upon failure", patients must be left wondering who is going to be affected by these necessary medical failures and hoping it won't be them.

However, Syed also observes, "Practice is about harnessing the benefits of learning from failure while reducing its cost." This leads to the logical conclusion that medical school and postgraduate medical training should offer an environment in which it is safe to fail – where we can mess up, no patient is harmed, and we learn the lessons for next time. The theory is sound, but our ability to implement it is limited by a single, central problem: the further through medical training we get, the more challenging the procedures become, the more complex the decisions we face, the greater the levels of responsibility and the more devastating the consequences of failure. As a result, clinical scenarios become harder to either simulate or to learn on the job without exposing patients to some degree of increased risk. In other words, the more senior we become in medicine, the harder it gets to progress safely.

Consider the tasks faced by medics at the bottom of the tree. When I started as a clinical medical student, the first procedure we learnt was phlebotomy. The hospital skills lab was set out with life-size model arms for us to practise on, each one complete with arteries and veins filled with artificial blood. Once we'd managed successfully with the models, we began practising on each other and by the end of the week we were tentatively taking our first blood samples on the wards. By the end of the year, we'd done dozens of blood tests, all the time learning from our mistakes, which resulted in nothing worse than a bruised arm for the patient and bruised egos for us.

This, then, was the ideal way of learning: a good simulation, a safe space to make mistakes and failures that were associated with minimal patient harm. Perhaps for this reason, most patients are perfectly happy to have a student do their blood test, often holding out their arm and declaring, "Well you've got to learn somehow, haven't you?" Some months later when we had progressed to inserting cannulas, an elderly woman had wobbly veins. I'd failed my first attempt. I suggested she might like the nurse to do it instead. "No, no, no dear," she insisted. "I want to see you win!" Her forbearance gave me the opportunity to learn instantly from my mistake. I picked a better vein, adjusted my technique and got the cannula into place.

When the potential harms are small, patients willingly volunteer to help us up the learning curve. However, as the complexity grows and the stakes get higher it becomes increasingly problematic for patients to take on this role, and medical professionals are less forthcoming regarding the extent to which a patient will be 'practised upon'. For example, when I began working in Intensive Care, I wanted to learn to insert central lines, a procedure that is associated with a long list of possible complications. Although I was fully supervised when I did my first ever central line insertion, with Nick, an Advanced Critical Care

Practitioner, displaying the patience of a saint and painstakingly talking me through every step of the process, there's no denying that the risk to the patient would have been lower if Nick had just done the line himself.

This issue is brought sharply into focus by considering the other extreme of the spectrum that begins with medical students taking blood – the most risk-fraught specialties, such as neurosurgery. In his bestselling book *Do No Harm*, the neurosurgeon Henry Marsh describes the problem as follows:

> It's one of the painful truths about neurosurgery that you only get good at doing the really difficult cases if you get lots of practice, but that means making lots of mistakes at first and leaving a trail of injured patients behind you.[39]

When I heard Marsh speak at Blackwell's Bookshop in Oxford in 2014, an audience member asked him how he decided when to let his juniors do the operating. He responded, almost sadly, "you have an ethical obligation to the patient in front of you, but also an ethical obligation to your juniors' future patients . . . and the two are utterly incompatible." Another audience member pushed him on how this incompatibility can be resolved in practice. He concluded that the best we can do is to have the consultant in the hospital pretty much all the time, providing close supervision and support.

It seems sensible that doctors learning new things should progress under the watchful guidance of expert clinicians, but there remains an inescapable truth: doctors never stop having to learn new things. And, as discussed in Chapter 1, there will always be a first time for doing a procedure or making an unsupervised decision. We will have to act independently at some stage. Furthermore, every time we progress up the medical ladder, we have tougher decisions to get right, a new level of challenge to meet and ever-present cognitive traps to fall into, meaning that the learning curve inevitably results in mistakes that pose a risk to patients. It has been said that those striving for high performance should remind themselves that even the greatest musicians must first play a lot of wrong notes. The trouble is, in medicine, a wrong note could be a tragedy. What's more, the wrong notes may not be audible immediately. We have to actively listen for them.

Hearing the Wrong Notes

The idea of 'feedback' for doctors usually conjures up images of meetings with supervisors, endless surveys in our inboxes or mandatory electronic forms that we are required to collect for an e-portfolio. As Kate Womersley and Katherine Ripullone wrote in the *BMJ*, "As a junior doctor, there's no escape from feedback"[40]. However, they also point out a systematic review published in the *BMJ* in 2010 that found "there is no evidence that workplace-based assessments lead to better performance, and limited evidence to support multi-score feedback"[41]. Speaking to numerous friends and colleagues, it is overwhelmingly clear that digital feedback forms and workplace-based assessments, whilst easily created, distributed and audited, have multiplied in volume to the point that they are widely regarded as little more than a tick-box exercise.

Instead, truly valuable feedback with the potential to improve our clinical thinking and reasoning, to help us decide better and to keep our patients safer, lies in the slow, incremental accumulation of discovering whether we got things wrong or right (or somewhere in-between). In *Nudge*, a book exploring human choices and decision-making, Professors Richard Thaler and Cass Sunstein say, "People make good choices in contexts in which they have experience, good information and prompt feedback . . . they do less well in contexts in which they are inexperienced and poorly informed, and in which feedback is slow or infrequent"[42]. Matthew Syed in *Black Box Thinking* similarly highlights the importance of feedback, commenting, "Without access to the error signal, one could spend years in training or in a profession without improving at all"[43].

In the same way that we should check back on our patients *during* a shift to see whether their treatment is working, and thus gain immediate feedback, we also need to seek them out in the following days to extend our period of follow-up. Obtaining this feedback on our clinical thinking and decision-making might happen routinely if we work a string of successive days on the same ward, but may not happen at all for patients we have clerked in 'front door' environments who are then admitted to any one of several different areas. This is problematic, since it is in the acute admissions setting that some of the most important diagnostic thinking and decision-making takes place. If we are to genuinely maximise our learning from the cases we are involved in, we need to find out what happened to our patients, to see whether our diagnosis was correct and whether the treatments we prescribed helped. This process might be anything from checking blood results after electrolyte replacement or seeing whether the radiologist's report on a chest X-ray matches our own interpretation, to reviewing a patient in person to get a better grasp of the natural history of their disease.

Unfortunately, junior doctors do not have allocated time in the busy rota for following patients up, so it has to be a proactive effort on our part. It is a shame that protected educational time is almost always reserved for didactic lecture-style teaching, where we will retain only a very small percentage of the content. In an *Emergency Medicine Journal* commentary on Adams and colleagues' research into junior doctors' clinical reasoning discussed in Chapter 1, Robert Lloyd argues that there should be protected time for case follow-up.[44] He comments,

> The transient nature of our patient encounters in the ED can lead to an 'out of sight, out of mind' culture, where we fail to follow up uncertain or particularly interesting cases. . . . This represents a glaring missed opportunity for learning, and the lack of diagnostic feedback potentially leads to the propagation of flawed clinical reasoning, particularly in inexperienced doctors.

Lloyd goes on to envision a system where hospital and departmental culture actively facilitates and encourages the seeking of meaningful feedback, with supervisors helping juniors to reflect on their learning. A supported and supervised setting of this kind probably represents the best way to discover what we have got wrong as well as what we have got right, where doctors with more experience can offer some perspective on mistakes and ensure mountains are not made from mole hills. Whilst this would be ideal, we should be prepared for the possibility of hearing wrong notes at a time that is not supervised, or ideal, and may be in the middle of a shift when we still have numerous other priorities to attend to.

The worst possible version of this, a scenario dreaded by doctors and nurses alike, is the crash bleep going off and announcing the impending or actual cardiac arrest of a patient you have been responsible for. In a horrifying moment, your heartbeat quickens, your stomach turns, your legs become jelly and your mind races as you run through the possibilities and wonder whether something you have done, or not done, has brought about this turn of events.

Two months into my time at the Small Hospital, I was upstairs on the first floor when the pager wailed and the voice announced, "Cardiac Arrest . . . AMU . . . Bed 14." I rushed back downstairs, through the pair of heavy double doors and into the unit to see the crash team assembled around the bed space of Alfred, a 74-year-old gentleman I had been looking after since the ward round that morning. Chest compressions were ongoing, the brutal reality of CPR leaving its marks on Alfred's lifeless body, and the rhythm on the monitor remained stubbornly non-shockable. My thoughts were in overdrive. How could this have happened? I had seen Alfred sat up drinking orange squash less than an hour earlier. What had I missed? I was sure I had done the jobs the consultant had asked me to. Meanwhile the resuscitation continued, without success, and when it became clear that Alfred could not be revived, the decision was taken to stop. Alfred had died.

I had been to cardiac arrests before, but never for one of my own patients, and certainly not for someone who had seemed to be doing so well just minutes beforehand. I was worried, and it must have shown, since Laura my SHO sat me down and explained that although she didn't know what had caused Alfred to die, she was sure it wasn't anything I was responsible for. As it turned out, nobody else was sure what had caused Alfred to die either and his family agreed to a post-mortem examination. Some weeks later Suzie from the bereavement office, who showered the new doctors with kindness and tea and biscuits through those cold winter afternoons, got in touch. She told me that Alfred had died from a ruptured thoracic aortic aneurysm – he had had a ticking time bomb in his chest, which we couldn't have known about. I hadn't done anything wrong.

Whilst the final, autopsy-proven feedback in Alfred's case had reassured me that I hadn't made a mistake, what about if we *have* done something wrong, causing actual or potential harm to the patient, when we *will* feel responsible? When we have caused an accidental emergency, how should we process and respond to this kind of unplanned but necessary feedback?

Error

Lying in bed one morning after a night shift, now several months into my first year of doctoring, I was struggling to sleep. It was warm and nearly summer, and I'd woken up mid-morning. Sleeping in the daytime had seemed easier in the winter, when it was cold and dark outside whether it was day or night, and you'd curl up into the duvet to leave the howling wind and the rest of the world outside. Breaking sleep hygiene recommendations straight away, I reflexively looked at my iPhone. Eoin, one of my colleagues and good friends from work, had messaged me:

> "I've just been to a peri-arrest call on the surgical ward . . . this guy had a potassium level of 8.2 and was really bradycardic . . .

he's a dialysis patient and someone had given him IV potassium overnight."

"Wow, really?" I responded. "I'm sure that wasn't me, and anyhow you'd have recognised my handwriting on the chart."

"No, I didn't look at the chart," he typed back. He texted me the patient's bed number.

Now I thought about it again and remembered – it *had* been me. I realised what I had done, and guilt and panic crashed over me as it dawned that I had just made a very serious mistake. My pulse was spiralling now, palpitations hammering in my chest.

I messaged Eoin again.

"I think he's going to be fine," he replied. "But critical care had to come, and the renal team took him for emergency dialysis."

Imagined images flooded into my head now, the medical emergency playing out in my mind's eye. The initial panic as the nurse found the patient profoundly bradycardic, his blood pressure so low as to be un-recordable. The buzzer being pulled, the alarm wailing, the crash team descending on the patient, emergency drugs being drawn up, temporary electrical pacing of the heart, the discovery of the potassium level and the risk-fraught transfer to the dialysis unit. All this had happened, because of me.

How could I have done this? I wracked my brains and recalled the start of the previous night. I'd been asked to cannulate a patient, an elderly man called Pascal who'd just been admitted. I'd checked the bloods. Low potassium at 2.8 mmol/L, so it needed replacing, I had thought. I had checked the kidney function – not great but kidneys working, I had thought. Now I realised my mistake – I had been hoodwinked by a set of post-dialysis bloods into thinking that Pascal's kidneys were working adequately. Now I could see that the clues had been there all along, his dialysis fistula obscured in the shadows of the darkening ward as I cannulated *the opposite arm*. I considered how Pascal was a renal patient who had had the misfortune to both end up on a surgical ward with abdominal pain that had no surgical cause, and to cross paths with me, a new doctor so utterly incompetent as to miss the fact that his kidneys were not functioning one iota. The fluid prescription I had written, which would have been routine and completely safe in almost any other patient, had very nearly killed him.

Eoin called me and began to apologise profusely for disturbing my sleeping between nights, but I quickly stopped him. If not the ideal way to hear these wrong notes, it was surely better than finding out in the middle of the subsequent night shift. I was glad he had told me. At least this way I had some time to try and get my thoughts together before heading back into the hospital for another night. But that was easier said than done. For the next 6 hours or so, I tossed and turned in the summer heat, disturbed by what I had done, falling in and out of a fitful slumber, until at last it was time to get up and trudge back to town and catch the bus to work.

Now I was nervous and afraid, dreading the impending moment when I would search for Pascal's name on the electronic records, silently praying to a God I don't believe in that the red "deceased" icon would not be staring back at me when I opened his file. It was a moment bizarrely reminiscent of other loading screens I'd faced down in the past, the seconds seeming an eternity as you await the downloading of something that you feel will change the course and direction of your life irreversibly. Eoin had said he thought Pascal would be ok, but a lot could have changed in the hours since then. Finally, the screen loaded. The location showed up as the renal ward – he wasn't dead.

That was all I needed to know for now, as I had the whole of the new night shift to get through. But how could I get through it? How could I make any decisions or take any action for the patients who needed me? How could I ever trust myself to prescribe anything again? Now more acutely aware of my blind spots than ever before, could I decide if I was competent to decide? I resolved to start slowly and build myself back up. I prescribed some paracetamol for a patient as the nurse asked, checking and double-checking their weight and liver function tests before doing so. Blimey. It was going to be a long night.

I was right – it was a long night, but not for the reasons I had thought. Incredibly, the time was going so slowly because there was almost nothing to do. The wards were settled, and the surgical admissions unit was similarly calm. On this night of all nights, when I was feeling helpless and paralysed and unable to make decisions, my luck was in and there were no decisions to make. I might have done a couple of cannulas, perhaps prescribed some codeine and reviewed one not very sick patient. The bleep stayed silent. This was so unusual that I bleeped myself to test if it was working. To this day, it remains the calmest night shift I have ever done. There have been just a handful of times in my life when things have worked out so perfectly that if I believed in God, I would have said it was divine intervention. Sometimes things seem like they are just meant to happen in a particular way.

However, at around 6.30 am my luck ended, and I was called to see a woman on the urology ward who was apparently bradycardic with an un-recordable blood pressure. Oh my word. Why were they calling me about this and not putting out a crash call? I was only 30 seconds away, so I hurried onto the ward to find the patient sitting up and talking (so her blood pressure obviously wasn't un-recordable), but her heart rate was indeed extremely slow, somewhere in the mid-20s. She looked ok enough, but I realised I was not in the frame of mind to attempt to sort this out. What mattered was the patient being properly reviewed, so I told the nurses to call a medical emergency. Her heart rate was low enough to justify it, after all.

As I had suspected, she wasn't that sick and it was small fry for the seniors who arrived to assist me, a problem easily resolved that they would have forgotten about by the time they were collapsing into bed at 10 am. My mind, on the other hand, went straight back to Pascal. The sun was up now and it was time for me to tell the consultant what I had done.

Duty

When the team ran through the list of patients at the morning handover meeting, Pascal's case was briefly mentioned and we were told his care had been taken over by renal medicine. A fresh wave of guilt washed over me, as I sat in the corner and wished the ground would open up beneath me. As the meeting ended and everyone got up to leave, I caught the consultant before he headed off to theatre and confessed that I had been responsible. He paused for a second, and then asked his registrar to carry on without him and prepare the first patient of the day for their operation. What came next was not what I had expected. "Do you want a cup of tea?" he asked. "I'm having one." He came back with two mugs and some breakfast muffins he had conjured from nowhere.

I had hoped he would not be too angry, but in the conversation that followed I was almost caught off guard by the degree of understanding and empathy he showed with regards to my mistake. I found myself wondering whether perhaps as a trainee surgeon he, or one of his close colleagues, had once cut something that was not supposed to be cut, or whether something had happened in the course of his own career to engender the calm and measured response he was now showing. Of course, I did not ask. In any case, surgeons are no strangers to the risks that human error poses to patients.

We agreed that I would submit an incident form against myself, which might result in an investigation, but this was not something I should worry about, he assured me. I did this the following day, triggering a process that ended a couple of weeks later with a short meeting with the Divisional Director for Surgery, and nothing more. "Don't beat yourself up too much," the Director implored as we went our separate ways.

There was one more thing to do before I could begin to move on from the mistake. In his report into the scandal at Mid Staffordshire NHS Foundation Trust, Sir Robert Francis wrote about "candour" amongst healthcare professionals, defining it as

> the volunteering of all relevant information to persons who have or may have been harmed by the provision of services, whether or not the information has been requested, and whether or not a complaint or a report about that provision has been made.[45]

This created a widespread and long overdue acknowledgement amongst doctors that when things go wrong, we need to tell the patient. It is the 'Duty of Candour'.

And so, before the start of the following night shift, I made my way down to the renal ward to find Pascal. Bizarrely, my ID card wouldn't open the door. Had the security people got wind of my incompetence and taken action to keep me away, to keep me from doing any more harm? Another doctor arrived and had the same problem. Probably not then. Eventually a ward sister let us both in, and I found Pascal in a bed by the window. He was still unwell – a nasty gastroenteritis that seemed to be the source of his 'non-surgical' abdominal pain – but he was stable. I pulled up a chair, and a vague look of recognition passed across his face. We chatted a short while about how he was doing. Eventually, when it could be avoided no longer, I said:

> Pascal – I need to tell you, the reason your heart started going so slowly the other day, the reason you became critically unwell, was because I prescribed that potassium, which you didn't need. It caused the potassium level to become much, much too high. I'm really sorry.

He stopped for a while, thoughts seeming to ripple across his furrowed brow. "It's ok," he responded. "Really, it is. You are young. I was very sick when I arrived on that ward, and you were trying to help. You thought that you were doing the right thing." I was amazed that he could be so philosophical when I had very nearly killed him. "And," he continued "I think that perhaps you have not looked after so many patients like me, with kidneys like mine, no?" He was right again, of course.

After some more time, I said goodbye and went to document our conversation in Pascal's medical notes, completing the 'Duty of Candour' requirements. I had been extremely grateful for my consultant's understanding, but with Pascal I knew I had been fortunate again. Other patients, or their families, would certainly have taken a different attitude towards what had happened. Pascal though, in his wisdom, had absolved me. With the weight on my shoulders a little lighter now, I went back upstairs to start the new night shift's work.

In the days and weeks that followed, my confidence slowly returned and I got back to, and then continued to progress beyond, my previous level of clinical practice. The mistake stayed with me, but I was able to start moving forwards. I hoped that in time more good than harm could come out of what had happened. I resolved to try to be kinder in my thoughts and less judgemental when I found patients who had received less than optimal care in our struggling hospital, to understand that everyone was trying their best in exceptionally trying circumstances, to not blame others as Pascal had not blamed me.

Amongst many, many smaller errors, Pascal's case was the one very significant mistake in my time as a new doctor. However, it seems certain that in the further years of training, and then practice as GPs or consultants, which lie ahead of us, there are other mistakes in waiting, both for me and for us all. The uncertainty and complexity we grapple with makes it this way. Professor James Reason, an industrial psychologist whose famous "Swiss Cheese Model" depicting a "cumulative act effect" ensured his position as an intellectual forefather of the patient safety field, underlined this point at the end of a BBC Radio 4 series discussing medical error. He reminded us, "It is sometimes said that there are only two kinds of doctor – those who have harmed a patient, and those who will harm a patient"[46]. If, then, it is a case of when and not if we will make mistakes, with or without significant patient harm, how should we process them, learn from them and make sense of our culpability?

Culpability

When things go wrong in healthcare, there is a tendency to immediately jump to the question of who is responsible for the mess we have found and to ask who is to blame. I have been guilty of this on more than one occasion, coming across patients who have been incorrectly treated and looking for an easy answer as to why, namely that Doctor so-and-so got it wrong. However, it should be self-evident that errors arising in complex systems have complex (and usually multi-faceted) origins. James Reason, writing in *A Life in Error: From Little Slips to Big Disasters*, points out that "when an organisational accident occurs, the key question is not who blundered, but how and why did the defences fail?"[47] Indeed, 16 years earlier in his 1997 book *Managing the Risks of Organisational Accidents*, Reason had put forward a "decision tree" for determining culpability for unsafe acts.[48] A simplified version is shown in Figure 2.1. In so doing, Reason offered not only an objective system for deciding whether an individual really was as culpable as they might first have seemed, but also a strategy for focusing in on the part of the system where defences against an error could be strengthened.

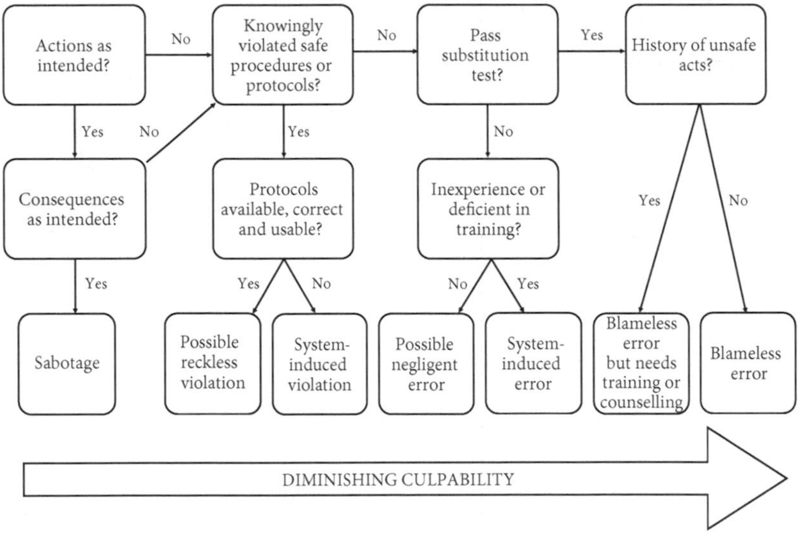

Figure 2.1 Decision Tree for Unsafe Acts Culpability (After James Reason, 1997.)

We can see the decision tree in action using my mistake with the potassium as an example. Starting at the top left-hand corner, we are asked, "Were the actions as intended?" Yes, I intended to prescribe the potassium, but (next question), no, the consequences were certainly *not* as intended. Then we are asked whether I "knowingly violated safe operating procedures?" (No again.)

The next question is a little more subjective: Would the error "Pass the substitution test?" The idea of the substitution test is to ask whether somebody of equivalent training, background and experience (in this case another new doctor) would have done the same thing, were they to have been substituted into my shoes in that same clinical scenario. It is similar to the "Bolam test" used in UK medical negligence law that asks whether the doctor fell below "the standard of the ordinary skilled man exercising and professing to have that special skill", although Reason's substitution test is notably more sympathetic to the reality of the prevailing situational and human factors. Many of my colleagues, as they tried to support me after the error, professed that they thought they could have made the same mistake, that "it could have been any one of us". But would they really have got it as wrong as I had, or were they just being nice? I'm sure the reality is somewhere in the middle – many wouldn't have made that particular error, but others may have done. Either way, the outcome of the decision tree looks relatively kindly on my mistake. If we deem the act of prescribing the potassium to have failed the substitution test, then I can certainly be classified as inexperienced, producing a verdict of a "system-induced error". If you decide that it passes the substitution test, we note that I did not have a "history of unsafe acts", giving a verdict of a "blameless error". In either case, the decision tree has moved our thinking on culpability some way beyond the simplistic blame culture logic of individual mistakes meaning individual culpability.

Thankfully, the medical profession is slowly taking steps away from a blame culture when it comes to mistakes, with many influential clinicians taking up Reason's mantle and advocating for systems-based analyses of medical errors. Scott Weingart is a Professor of Emergency Medicine in New York, who has been made world-famous amongst critical care doctors by his EMCrit podcast. Speaking to Dr Andrew Davies on the *Mastering Intensive Care* podcast in July 2019, Weingart powerfully argued for an understanding of clinician errors that resembles the philosophy of Reason's decision tree:

> When we do make a mistake there's a tendency to beat ourselves up. There's an idea in most people's heads of libertarian free will . . . that given the exact same set of circumstances we could have behaved differently. But that's an absolute fallacy . . . no one who actually understands this stuff thinks that given the exact same set of circumstances you could have done anything different. Now think that through – it means that when you do make an error, as long as you weren't coming to work drunk, as long as you have not been slacking for the last ten years . . . if you were playing the game as well as you could and there was an error, there was absolutely nothing that could have happened differently than that, and due to all the other circumstances around you – multiple patients, someone happened to distract you at just the wrong moment – there's nothing that could have been done differently.[49]

In a system where discussions following significant events have traditionally boiled down to asking, "What could you have done differently?" the assertion that we should evaluate errors from the starting point of, "There's *nothing* that could have been done differently" is a radical one. It is hard to escape the mindset that someone could have acted differently, calculated that dose correctly, called for help sooner or made a safer decision. Why didn't they just get it right? Can it really be the case that nobody could have acted differently and prevented the error?

Yes, it can. Just as Reason's decision tree analyses an individual's actions taken in that exact situation at that exact moment in time, Weingart is repeatedly clear on the condition that "given the exact same set of circumstances" nothing could have been different. The adage attributed to the Greek philosopher Heraclitus of Ephesus that "No man ever steps in the same river twice, for it's not the same river and he's not the same man" is useful here. Someone with the benefit of hindsight (the medical retrospectoscope!) could not be the same person, because they have gained knowledge or understanding from the error, and they could not stand in the same river, because that would involve time travel. From a linguistic perspective, it is the choice of modal verb that matters; we *would* have done something differently (had we known), we *should* have done something differently (of course), but in those exact circumstances we *could* not have done anything differently, since that was how the events played out. Rather than "que sera sera" (what will be will be), it is a case of "what was, was" or "what happened, happened".

This view of medical error has several important implications. Firstly, it provides a roadmap for doctors to discuss errors both with supervisors and within their teams, suggesting that asking "What could have been done differently?" could be replaced with a more open, conversational "debriefing" style of interaction. I first came across the idea of debriefing during a training course for delivering high-fidelity medical simulations. Debriefing fundamentally differs from giving feedback in that it seeks to guide and support the learners' own discussion of events, rather than didactically raising specific positive and negative points.

One popular model used in simulation-based education is the 'Diamond Debrief', which moves through phases of description ("What happened?"), analysis ("Why did you respond in that way?" or "Why did you take that action?") and application ("What would you do if you found yourself in a similar situation again?").[50] The aim is to spend proportionally more time in the middle analytical phase than in the initial description phase or the closing application phase, giving the 'Diamond' structure to the session. This kind of approach seems to accept without judgement that events occurred the way they did, before constructively elucidating the useful learning from any mistakes. Once we shift away from a blame culture in healthcare and start from the position that the individuals involved were almost certainly neither murderous nor drunk nor stupid, we are in a better position to ask the key analysis phase question of why the actions taken seemed to make sense at the time. We can begin to understand the multitude of educational, training, environmental, situational, team and patient factors that aligned to allow for the error to happen. We can talk about why the system's defences failed, about each of the holes in the Swiss cheese and why on the occasion in question they tragically fell into line.

The second key implication of Reason's theory of diminishing culpability is that it offers a route away from damaging mental self-admonishment for clinicians who have made an error. When the vast majority of errors fall into the categories of "system-induced error" or "blameless error" at the right-hand side of the decision tree, helping someone to appreciate that their role was only one part of an error chain, and that their possible re-training or further education is only one part of the required solution, is likely to ease the individual burden considerably. And we know what a burden it can be. Pending investigations following an error or a patient complaint have been cited as contributory factors in multiple physician suicides, a topic we will return to in Chapter 6. When things go wrong for hard-working doctors whose sense of self-worth is often tied, to a greater or lesser extent, to the quality of their clinical work, the mental downward spiral can be dramatic. We are at risk of becoming what has been described as "the second victim"[51].

I regularly thank my lucky stars that Pascal did not die, that he was saved from my error by the intervention of experienced medical doctors and critical care. Although he remained unwell with his presenting condition and advanced comorbidities, I am grateful that he survived his encounter with me, with my inexperience, with my clinical naivety, and that he did not come to any lasting harm by my hand. I am grateful primarily for him and for his family, but also, selfishly, for myself. I am genuinely scared to contemplate the path I would have begun to tread had his nurse reached him much later, had he gone on to have a cardiac arrest and to die. The 48 hours of mental turmoil until it became apparent he would be ok could so nearly have been 48 days, or 48 weeks.

Martin Bromiley is an airline pilot who became a leader and campaigner for understanding human factors in healthcare following the death of his wife Elaine after a nightmarish "Can't Intubate, Can't Oxygenate" anaesthetic scenario. Asked on the *Mastering Intensive Care* podcast about the somewhat cynical view that healthcare is unlike aviation because if the 'plane' crashes in healthcare the pilot will not also die, Bromiley remarked poignantly,

> There is a newer generation of doctors who understand the impact of a fatal error . . . on themselves. If you put your hand on your heart and think about people you know who have made fatal errors in healthcare, the impact on them is as good as dying.[52]

It is a mark of his emotional intelligence and empathy that, as the bereaved husband of a wife who died because of medical error and healthcare systems failure, Bromiley champions the mental wellbeing of clinicians that have made these kinds of mistakes.

Importantly though, adopting a more nuanced and balanced understanding of our role when things have gone wrong is not a 'Get Out of Jail Free' card. It is not a view of medical error to be endorsed on the basis that it conveniently absolves us of responsibility. When things have gone wrong, we will always share in and carry responsibility for what has happened, because we are trusted so intensely. Patients' trust, as they struggle for breath in the Emergency Department, share some hidden fraction of their evolving sadness in a consulting room or hold out their cannulated hand to be put to sleep for an operation, is why medicine will never be "just a job". It matters a lot, and it is right that we feel responsible.

However, I wonder whether the important distinction to be made is that between culpability and responsibility. Beyond a period of sensible self-reflection after an error, focusing too much on a personal sense of culpability, wondering repeatedly, "If only I'd done x, y or z differently" is not, in the end, much use to anyone. On the other hand, understanding our own position in an error-chain, amongst the multitude of factors that allowed for the error to occur, should create the conditions for improvement to become possible, handing us back the responsibility to gain meaningful learning from the event and to think about systems-level change. Scott Weingart commented,

> Blaming yourself . . . is a useless and counter-productive situation. Now, *use* the error, to spur you to go further – to read about that, to think about it, to ask yourself 'What am I going to put in place to make sure that particular error doesn't happen again?' But to spend even one moment berating yourself for 'Why didn't I?' is bullshit.

The ball is in our court. What we do with it is our responsibility.

Wrongs and Rights

In this chapter, we have acknowledged the inevitable errors associated with learning curves in medicine, seeing that whilst the challenge for individuals is to proactively seek the error signal in order to improve, the challenge for organisations and institutions is to instigate systems and supervision to ensure that the risks and harms to patients are kept to an absolute minimum. We have also seen that even outside the obvious learning curves of practising new technical procedures or prescribing new drugs, the complexity faced by new doctors (and less new ones) means that the potential for mistakes is always there, producing both near misses and harrowing instances of patient harm. When these adverse events do occur, the opportunity both for individual clinicians to recover and for future risks to be mitigated depends largely on where an organisation sits on the spectrum from blame culture to just culture. Fortunately for new doctors entering the profession, there are reassuring signs that institutional thinking is beginning to shift in the right direction, thanks to the accelerating work of the patient safety movement over the past two decades.

Importantly, learning in patient safety should not only arise from healthcare going wrong. It is becoming increasingly recognised that clinical learning and improvements should also be gained from when things go well. James Reason commented in *A Life in Error*, "Human beings can be heroes as well as hazards, a fact that is largely ignored in a research methodology triggered primarily by the occurrence of adverse events"[53]. In the next chapter, we consider what we can learn about keeping our patients safe from the everyday work of new doctors getting things right. However, the bottom of the medical chain can be a tough place to take action from, so we also consider how we can best advocate for patients when we are playing the right notes, but struggling to be heard.

"The real voyage of discovery consists not in seeking new lands but in seeing with new eyes."

Marcel Proust, *A la recherche du temps perdu*

3

HEALTHY SAFETY

HOW CAN NEW DOCTORS GET THINGS RIGHT?

The Team Works

Summer was beginning to roll into view, and we had somehow already made it to the third rotation of the year, which was general surgery. Time flies when you're having fun, but also when you're on a full-time doctor's rota, it turned out. The weeks were rapidly turning into months, which accumulated behind us. It was just past 8 pm on a humid Saturday evening. Night handover was approaching and I was parked behind the desk, trying to get together a list of the patients with outstanding blood results to chase. It was slow going. My brain was addled, and there were more than 80 inpatients on the list, spread across seven different wards. I really needed this shift to be done with and to get home. Sanith, one of my pals who was also on the general surgery rotation, arrived for the start of the night shift. "Alright mate," he beamed as he walked in. "Hope the day's not been too bad?"

"Well . . ." I began, gesturing at the state of the list in front of me.

Suddenly, the crash buzzer started wailing. I jumped up with a start, trying to see where it was coming from. It was somewhere in Bay 3. As a healthcare assistant started dialling 2222 on the nearby desk phone, Sanith and I followed the nurses into the bedspace, where we saw a middle-aged woman called Julie lying unconscious, eyes rolling back in her head, foam bubbling from her mouth, all four of her limbs shaking violently. Julie had returned to the ward from her planned gallbladder operation earlier that evening, but now she seemed to be having what looked like a generalised tonic-clonic seizure. I glanced left and right, looking but knowing what I would see. We were the only doctors there.

It had already been an exhausting day, but the adrenaline surge from the crash call snapped me into action.

"Ok, let's pull the bed out, and take the headboard off."

Before I even had time to release the brake pedal, two of the ward nurses, Leah and Sophie, had done as I'd asked, so I moved round to the head of Julie's bed.

"Let's raise the bed a little higher. Leah, please can I have the suction?"

Again, almost immediately, the nurses placed the suction in my hand. The voice of one of the clinical tutors from medical school played in my head: "Remember, suction only what you can see." The vacuum from the plastic tube was working well and I removed the worst of the foam from the front of Julie's mouth. What was more, the seizing looked like it was stopping, thank goodness. But almost as soon as her limbs became still, Julie started snoring.

"Let's give 15 L/minute of oxygen via the non-rebreathe mask," I decided. Once more, the team was moving in sync around us. The mask was passed to me, with someone already having attached it to the oxygen socket in the wall. I inflated the reservoir bag and pulled the elastic cords over the back of Julie's head. A pulse oximeter was simultaneously being fitted to Julie's finger, giving a reading of just 85%. I opened her airway with a jaw-thrust manoeuvre, which seemed to stop the snoring noises. The oxygen saturations began to improve. For the first time in my life, I was having to do some basic airway management – independently.

Keep carrying on. Airway first. Breathing next. With me tied up at the head of the bed, Sanith now took the lead.

"Sophie, please will you do a full set of observations?" he asked.

Sanith quickly examined Julie's breathing, watching the equal rise and fall of her chest, percussing with two fingers and listening with his stethoscope to confirm that there was air entry on both sides. How long had it been since the medical emergency call had been put out? As the entirety of our focus was narrowed on Julie, time seemed to be going into slow motion around us. Surely the registrar, the SHOs and the critical care nurses would have to arrive soon? Nobody came, so we carried on.

Breathing was ok. Circulation next. The blood pressure Sophie had measured was 132/75 mmHg, with a pulse rate of 68. Ok, fine. What comes next? D is for 'Disability', including level of consciousness, which was clearly the major issue here. Despite her limbs having stopped shaking, Julie hadn't woken up. People who have had a seizure are usually very tired and confused when it ends, but they should begin to regain consciousness. Julie, on the other hand, remained completely unconscious. We had assessed and managed her airway, breathing and circulation and the seizing had stopped, but for some reason she was not waking up. My clinical tutor's voice returned in my head. ABCD . . . and DEFG, "Don't Ever Forget Glucose!"

At that point Aidan, one of the medical registrars, and the crash team came rushing into the bay. They all looked red-faced, hot and flustered. We later found out that there had been three almost simultaneous crash calls across the hospital, so despite the narrowing of our perception we hadn't been entirely wrong about the passage of time. We had been managing Julie on our own for slightly longer than we otherwise would have done. Sanith handed over the story.

> "Have we checked the blood glucose?" Aidan asked. Leah promptly did. It was dangerously low, at 2.2 mmol/L.
>
> "200 mLs of 10% dextrose?" I suggested. We gave the IV bolus, correcting the blood sugar level to well above 5 mmol/L. However, Julie still did not wake up.

I stayed where I was, maintaining her airway, my hands sweating in the hastily grabbed gloves that were a size too small and starting to ache with my inexpert and unpractised technique. A critical care nurse assisted me and inserted a nasopharyngeal airway, reducing the need for the jaw thrust. Through all this, Julie remained unconscious.

Things were rapidly becoming more serious now, a realisation that coincided with the arrival of the ICU registrar, closely followed by her consultant. The ICU team assumed control of the situation, and when Julie failed to respond to the medications they tried, they made the decision to intubate her immediately, on the ward. Once safely asleep and attached to a portable ventilator, she was transferred to the unit.

Aidan took Sanith and me aside. "Well done, you two," he told us. "You were managing nicely on your own there before we arrived." We were grateful to know that we had done all we could and done what our training had prepared us for, but that gratitude was surpassed the following day when we heard that Julie was awake, extubated and was going to be ok. She left ICU with a diagnosis of hypoglycaemic non-convulsive status epilepticus. We couldn't have known what the diagnosis was when we first responded to the crash buzzer, but working as a team with the experienced nurses had enabled us to keep Julie safe and to get things right.

A Second Frame

When considering how doctors get things right, it would be tempting to simply look at the various factors that help us manage in a crisis – the self, team and environmental elements that we handled well when faced with an acutely ill patient. "What allowed for things to go so well?" we might ask afterwards, as we pat ourselves on the back. If we can learn from these aspects, won't we have found the key to getting things right? Not entirely. Although human factors that affect emergency performance are essential to understand and will be discussed later in this chapter, the management of clinical crises is only one part of the picture. Indeed, in some cases these crises might not have arisen if things had gone right at an earlier, non-emergency stage. Prevention is better than cure.

At the end of Chapter 2, I highlighted James Reason's comment that "human beings can be heroes as well as hazards", but it is the second part of his statement, referring to this being "largely ignored in a research methodology triggered primarily by adverse events"[54], which is particularly important. Never events, adverse events, near misses and critically unwell ward patients like Julie are all highly salient, sticking in our minds in part because they are relatively rare. So, we investigate them, do research about them and try to learn from them. However, the heroics Reason alludes to are not our efforts at these times of crisis, but the everyday actions that are common, and consequently unrecognised and under-appreciated. Could the secret to getting things right lie hidden in the everyday that is *not* at the forefront of our brains, in the positive points that are missed and don't even register?

In an agenda-setting white paper published in 2015, Professors Erik Hollnagel, Robert Wears and Jeffrey Braithwaite elaborated two distinct perspectives on patient safety, which they termed Safety-1 and Safety-2.[55] The traditional view of safety as the absence of accidents and incidents is the Safety-1 perspective, where healthcare practitioners and the systems we work in aim for as few things as possible to go wrong. This is the perspective of the NHS England patient safety definition that we encountered in Chapter 1. From the Safety-2 perspective, on the other hand, safety is defined as the situation in which as many things as possible go right. In a world focused on Safety-1, we hope to high heaven that we do not get things wrong and are then reactive in trying to learn from the errors when an adverse event does occur. But in a world that includes Safety-2, we proactively try to learn all the time from the frequent everyday things that go right.

The three professors suggest that all clinical outcomes lie somewhere on a normal distribution that describes the relationship between a given outcome and the likelihood of it occurring. In this model, outcomes that are entirely as planned or as expected lie at the origin and are the most frequent, whilst the tails of the distribution are the rarest outcomes: disasters such as never events on the far-left hand side and "positive surprises" such as early completion of work or unexpected patient recoveries on the far right-hand side. The traditional Safety-1 viewpoint, it is argued, has historically only been interested in the left-hand tail of this distribution, meaning that the frequently occurring planned outcomes or unexpectedly positive outcomes represent an untapped resource for learning.

Why do we neglect the positive outcomes and focus on learning predominantly from the negative? When a patient's outcome is as expected or better than expected, we say to ourselves something along the lines of, "We're doctors, this is our job, we're supposed to make people better. Nothing to see here." We tend to view most things on the right-hand side of that distribution as the status quo. But when something does not go as planned, even if it's just an unexpectedly difficult case and the patient isn't harmed, we perceive the outcome as negative. And if a mistake does cause actual patient harm, the event strikes to the core of how we see ourselves, of who we think we are. It can feel like a disaster.

The predictable response to doctors being overly focused on their mistakes would be to attribute it to Type-A personality traits such as being ambitious, status-conscious and perfectionist. "You're all perfectionists!" they'll say. "No wonder you're all about the mistakes. That's how you got past the competition to get into medical school in the first place." The logical extension of this argument, they'll continue, is that if only we would be a little less hard on ourselves and see the positive outcomes as being better than status quo, we could have a shot at learning within the Safety-2 framework when things have gone right. But Type-A personality traits are not the whole story.

In fact, the discrepancy in the psychological importance we attach to relatively negative, compared with relatively positive, outcomes has its foundations in a deep-rooted cognitive bias called loss aversion. Back in our ancestors' days as hunter–gatherers, the mental shortcuts and heuristics that give rise to potentially damaging cognitive biases were adaptive, highly functional traits that increased your odds of survival. When you heard twigs snapping in the undergrowth at night, it was a good thing to make some assumptions, reach a snap judgement and enact a quick decision. It was evolutionarily sensible for the human brain to prioritise threat avoidance ahead of approaching opportunities for possible gains. Richard Thaler summarises in *Misbehaving: The Making of Behavioural Economics* that "roughly speaking losses hurt about twice as much as gains make you feel good"[56].

Back in the world of medicine, this is why clinical 'losses' stick in our minds so much more. When patients' lives are at stake, our loss aversion bias is dominant. "We don't remember the countless times we got it right," my friend Kathy observed when I asked for her reflections on cases she had been involved with since qualifying. The positive value doesn't seem to register. By contrast, it is the profoundly negative psychological value we accrue when things have gone wrong that underlies our predilection for the Safety-1 perspective of aiming for the absence of accidents and incidents. But is this not entirely appropriate? It is the patients who adverse events happen to. We focus on Safety-1 to protect them, not to shield ourselves from negative psychological value. Isn't a healthy dose of negative psychological value just what's needed to focus some minds and prevent errors from happening again?

The first thing to say is that the Safety-2 perspective is not supposed to be a replacement way of thinking. It remains essential that we utilise Safety-1 constructively and learn the lessons when things do go wrong. It should continue to come first. Safety-2 is an *addition*, an alternative lens with which to view the problem, an opportunity that has the potential to offer new insights. Crucially, learning from things going right within Safety-2 is not about de-prioritising adverse events in order to blindly focus on happier outcomes, but is instead about building understanding of how things usually function correctly, in order to elucidate which parts of that process didn't happen on the occasion that something went wrong.

New doctors must aim not only to avoid making mistakes but also to get things right as often as possible. How can we make this happen? Hollnagel, Wears and Braithwaite write,

> Things do not go right because people behave as they are supposed to, but because people can and do adjust what they do to match the conditions of work. The challenge for safety improvement is . . . to understand how performance usually goes right in spite of the uncertainties, ambiguities, and goal conflicts that pervade complex work conditions.

They are talking about the benefits of flexibility, adaptability and critical thinking, which are important traits when we find ourselves in a 'VUCA' (Volatile, Uncertain, Complex and Ambiguous) environment. In the rest of this chapter, we will explore a range of individual, team and organisational factors that can affect our chances of getting things right. What can we learn about the hidden everyday aspects that might underlie our successes? Firstly, we will start with the compelling case for trying to be the nicest person in the hospital. As one ICU registrar phrased it, "The single most important human factor is just don't be a jerk."

Civility Saves Lives

It goes without saying that we should all be kind and polite to our colleagues. However, aside from the clear moral obligation to treat other people with kindness, there is also a convincing body of evidence telling us that civil behaviour is fundamental to getting things right. Much of the original research into this topic was conducted in the business sector, but very similar findings have subsequently been produced in healthcare. This important body of work has been highlighted in the UK by the "Civility Saves Lives" campaign, which was started by a group of healthcare professionals in the West Midlands. One of this group, Emergency Medicine consultant Chris Turner, said in his TEDxExeter talk titled "When Rudeness in Teams Turns Deadly" that "it looks like, for competent teams, the single most important factor determining the outcome of that team is how we treat each other"[57].

Civility is the opposite of rudeness (or incivility), which could take the form of interrupting, talking over or undermining someone, aggression, shouting or belittling behaviour. Notably, there is no single, fixed standard for civil behaviour between individuals, meaning that we need to remain aware of how those around us might be feeling. In her book *Mastering Civility: A Manifesto for the Workplace*, Professor Christine Porath explains, "Incivility is in the eyes of the recipient. It varies not just by individual but also by culture, generation, gender, industry, and organization. What you consider uncivil may not be the same thing your boss considers uncivil"[58]. This does make achieving civility begin to sound very complex, and like it could be a knotty problem. Actually, Porath's explanation is something that most of us probably already live by; we know intuitively that the level of volume and shouting that is permissible between teammates on a football or hockey field would be totally unacceptable between teammates in the office. Achieving civility across the board just means applying this same logic where there are more subtle distinctions to be made.

Christine Porath, working alongside her colleague Christine Pearson, found in surveys of 800 employees and managers across 17 industries that experiencing incivility affected people in ways including (but not limited to) 48% intentionally reducing their work effort, 80% losing work time worrying about the incident, 66% admitting to a decline in their performance and 25% taking their frustrations out on customers.[59] What about in healthcare teams, where the "customers" caught up in these effects are our patients?

There is plenty of observational data to suggest that incivility could have grave consequences. For example, in 2008, Rosenstein and O'Daniel published research that surveyed 4530 participants working in healthcare on the West Coast in the United States, of whom 67% agreed that disruptive behaviours they had witnessed were associated with adverse events, while 71% associated uncivil behaviour with medical errors.[60] Shockingly, 27% thought that the disruptive behaviours they had seen were linked with patient mortality. Survey results do not prove causation, of course, since there could be any number of hidden factors explaining the observations. However, recent high-quality randomised trials have solidified the link between incivility and risking patient safety.

Researchers at Tel Aviv University in Israel conducted a randomised, double-blind trial on the effect of rudeness in NICU teams in a simulated scenario involving the recognition and management of necrotising enterocolitis and then cardiac tamponade (as a complication of a leaking central line) in a pre-term infant.[61] Teams were randomised to receive either mildly rude comments about their clinical performance, or neutral (control) comments from an observing foreign expert on "team reflexivity in medicine". The teams on the receiving end of the rudeness were marked significantly lower on both diagnostic and procedural performance by three independent judges, effects that further analysis revealed could best be explained by reduced information-sharing and reduced help-seeking, respectively. Think back to the Johari Window in Figure 1.2 (Chapter 1). It seems as though just a few rude comments were enough to prevent the team successfully information sharing and expanding their 'arena' of useful and actionable information known to the whole team. Similarly, the psychological insult from the rudeness seemed to prevent people from asking for help with procedures when they needed it. In this particular simulated scenario, one of the procedures was pericardiocentesis, drawing fluid away from the pericardial sack surrounding the pre-term infant's heart. The consequences of incivility could hardly be more serious.

In another high-quality study, Katz and colleagues randomised anesthesiology residents participating in a simulated operative crisis involving occult haemorrhage to work with either a rude surgeon or a polite surgeon.[62] Of those teamed up with a polite surgeon, 91% performed as expected in the crisis and passed the simulation, whereas only 64% of those working with a rude surgeon did so. Despite this enormous effect size, there was no significant difference in the residents' self-reported performance, using a Likert scale. Even when we are the direct targets of incivility, we may be blind to its impact on our performance. Furthermore, rudeness exacerbates judgement biases, something that Cooper and colleagues highlight as being "fundamentally different from suboptimal performance"[63]. Cooper's group showed in a series of experiments involving medical diagnosis that rudeness worsens anchoring bias, which is the tendency to inappropriately fixate on a single point of information when forming a judgement and is thought to be by far the single most common cognitive bias in medicine.[64]

As if all this wasn't enough, incivility affects everyone who is close enough to witness it, even if they weren't the target of the original rudeness. Like a virus spreading from person to person, negative emotions *and the negative behaviours that triggered them* can rapidly spread through a group, an effect known as social contagion. Shoulders drop and heads turn away, as colleagues become uncomfortable in the presence of incivility. It's not just that they feel bad about what they're seeing. The witnesses themselves exhibit a 20% decrease in performance, and a 50% decrease in their willingness to help others. These are not trivial effects. In busy, high-pressure environments such as the ED or an acute admissions unit, the rudeness of just one person could affect the performance of dozens of colleagues around them, compromising their ability to deliver safe and compassionate care. The behaviours spread as well as the emotions. Those who witness incivility are more likely to subsequently behave poorly towards others, especially if the incivility came from a senior colleague. In this way, the problem can spread exponentially.

One element of the civility problem that new doctors are particularly vulnerable to is the veil of anonymity. The most junior doctors on clinical teams are often tasked to telephone colleagues from other departments with specific queries that need a specialist opinion. At least, the queries should be specific, but this is not always the case if the new doctor hasn't fully understood the clinical question and what exactly his or her consultant wanted to know. Usually this is because nobody took the time to explain it to them. Unfortunately, this exacerbates the major power imbalance when it comes to the phone call, with very junior doctors calling senior registrars or consultants, some of whom can be much ruder or more disrespectful on the phone than they ever would be in person. "I've had a terrible day!" one new doctor told me. "I had to call three different specialties and they all either thought it was a stupid question, made me feel like I was an idiot or refused to help at all. One of them wouldn't even tell me their name." Hiding behind the veil of anonymity, refusing junior colleagues even the basic courtesy of properly introducing yourself, is a hallmark of incivility that I sadly also had experienced.

When I was an Intensive Care SHO on the University Spaceship, I arrived for the start of one night and immediately had the sense that it was going to be a difficult shift. In her book *The Courage to Care*, Christie

Watson writes, "All hospital departments have their own beats and melodies and, if you listen carefully enough, you can hear them and work out what kind of shift it will be"[65]. She is right. With time in any placement, you develop an innate sense for the situation on your unit or ward, a sense for whether the preceding day or night shift you are arriving to relieve has been calm or horrendous or anywhere in-between. It must be the subconscious brain recognising and combining the tell-tale signs: the quiet or the bleeping of the alarms, the measured or frenetic pace of activity, the familiar friendly faces or the presence of new and unknown specialty teams called urgently to assist. On this particular evening, I had the strong feeling that the night would be difficult from the start.

Within an hour of the night handover, things were indeed kicking off. One patient who had been extubated that day was looking likely to need re-intubation, another was hyperkalaemic and would need a new central line for renal replacement therapy if it couldn't be medically managed, and another was becoming delirious and attempting to rip out his NG tube, central line and urinary catheter. On top of that, my registrar had been called down to ED resus to attend multiple trauma calls whilst we were still trying to do the night ward round. Additionally, the daytime team had asked me to make sure I called the general surgical registrar about the CT abdomen result for Mr Jablonski in Bed 14, which had shown a small but noticeable perforation in his small bowel. We needed to know if something should be done about it overnight.

I tried several times, at around 15-minute intervals, to bleep the surgical registrar, but got no answer. Mr Jablonski was stable enough for now, but the experienced nurse looking after him and I agreed that we really needed to know – we couldn't just ignore the radiology report of the bowel perforation, which itself stated, "I suggest seeking a surgical opinion." Besides, our own daytime ICU team had specifically asked me to call them. How would it look if we hadn't done that and Mr Jablonski became dangerously unwell? I gave it one final go, bleeping two different numbers provided by the switchboard operator. Still nothing. I couldn't carry on like this all evening. Sooner rather than later one of the other patients was going to need our full attention, so if Mr Jablonski's bowel was a problem, we had to know. When you are genuinely getting no response from a bleep, the (rare) next step is to 'over-bleep' that doctor. I called the surgical consultant.

"Hello, my name is Luke Austen, I'm one of the ICU SHOs. Please could I ask your advice about . . ."

"What, it's quarter past eleven, why are you calling me?"

"I'm sorry to bother you, I bleeped the surgical registrar but wasn't getting any response. It's about . . ."

"No, he always answers."

"I'm sorry, I did try a number of times. We have a critical care patient here called Mr . . ."

"This is ridiculous, what's this about?"

"We have a patient called Mr Jablonski . . . his CT scan shows a bowel perforation."

"Oh yeah him."

"My registrar asked me to discuss with the surgical team whether the CT finding needs to be acted on."

"Oh him! Him! We saw that scan hours ago! It's fine. Why are you calling me about this? It's totally inappropriate."

"I'm sorry to have troubled you, but he's a critical care patient and the radiologists did advise a discussion with surgery. I was asked to call your team and your registrar wasn't answering."

"But this CT scan is fine, we saw it hours ago! It's past eleven at night, why are you calling me?"

"We didn't know a decision had been made. There's nothing written in the notes. Nobody's come to see him or called us."

"This is all irrelevant! Totally irrelevant! Why are you calling me? It's very inappropriate."

"I'm sorry you feel that way. I need to write in the notes that we've discussed Mr Jablonski's case, please could I have your name for the notes?"

> "No! You can't have my name! This is all very inappropriate!"
> I hung up.

I was seething. I had only been a qualified doctor for 14 months, it was a lot of responsibility being on the ICU, and I needed my full energy focused on the multiple unwell patients on the unit. With my registrar tied up downstairs in ED and our Advanced Critical Care Practitioner alongside her to look after the patients she'd had to intubate that night, I'd need to anticipate the potential problems and fetch another registrar from the next-door ICU if any of our patients deteriorated. I really didn't have spare bandwidth to deal with this guy's rudeness. Why should I have to keep apologising for my own existence? I was only doing what my seniors had asked. Why should I have to put up with it?

I hit zero on the desk phone and called back the switchboard operator.

> "Hello, please could you tell me from the rota the name of the surgical consultant you just put me through to?"
> "Sure. Let me see. It was Mr Smith."

In the morning, once handover was done, I emailed our ICU consultant on-call and the consultant in charge of ICU, and complained.

Even as the most junior member of the team, you should be able to make phone calls to any seniors you need to in order to keep patients safe, without fear of being belittled or experiencing rudeness of any kind. Each individual, medical team, department and hospital has a responsibility to foster a culture where nothing less is expected, and nothing less is tolerated. Civility is not an end in itself, but a permissive factor that enables the kind of communication, creativity and critical thinking required for staff to appropriately adjust what they are doing in response to the needs of the complex clinical environment – this is the mode of success elaborated by Hollnagel, Wears and Braithwaite that we discussed earlier. It is no exaggeration to say that the way in which we treat each other is safety critical. Insisting upon a civil work environment is also a key part of achieving a broader team and institutional climate in which people, no matter how junior, are empowered to act in the best interests of their patients. This is the aim of achieving "psychological safety".

The Fearless Hospital

I first heard the term 'psychological safety' in the context of simulation-based education, where I understood the term to simply mean, "What happens in the Sim room stays in the Sim room." We were aiming for a situation where participants would feel able to express half-formed ideas, admit to not knowing something and make mistakes in a safe environment, without fearing that their performance would be gossiped about on the other side of those four walls. In fact, the type of psychological safety we wanted in the artificial Sim room environment has much in common with the psychological safety that is necessary for individuals and teams to get things right in the real world.

"Psychological safety is broadly defined as a climate in which people are comfortable being and expressing themselves," writes Harvard Professor of Leadership and Management Amy Edmondson in her book *The Fearless Organization*.[66] "More specifically," she continues, "when people have psychological safety at work, they feel comfortable sharing concerns and mistakes without fear of embarrassment or retribution." In the research that led Edmondson to coin the term and formally delineate the concept of psychological safety, she noticed that error rates were paradoxically higher in what were objectively higher performing teams, as judged by blinded and independent assessors. She realised that the higher performing teams had a group culture and climate in which members felt able to report mistakes, leading to their apparently elevated error counts. This hidden ingredient that facilitated the raising of issues and reporting of things going wrong was psychological safety. In the long term, feeling able to speak up helped these teams get things right and perform at a higher level.

Crucially, the level of psychological safety is something that varies not only between organisations, but within them too. In hospitals there are layers upon layers of subcultures within cultures, with the possibility of very different interpersonal environments for the various wards, units, teams, specialties or professions. The attitudes and behaviours of only one or a small number of individuals can dramatically alter levels of psychological safety within these groups, particularly when those people are highly placed within the institutional hierarchy.

As a new doctor on the surgical rotation, I worked with one consultant who created an environment around him that was the opposite of psychologically safe. Let's call him Mr Howard. Mr Howard was not civil. He was rude to his team and rude about the patients we were looking after. He was often moody and temperamental, unpredictably swinging from joviality to obvious irritation and grumpiness. In handover meetings, which are supposed to be a time for passing on key clinical information, he frequently appeared disinterested and would be on his iPhone when the most junior team members were speaking about their patients. Furthermore, he had a reputation for quizzing the new doctors at the end of their night shifts clerking on the SAU, and then openly criticising their slightest mistakes in front of the entire room. He was then manipulative in overly and overtly praising a different doctor, deliberately highlighting the contrast with the team member he had just criticised. "He made me feel so small and like I was so stupid," one colleague told me. "I felt like I could never become a good doctor after that. He really made me cry the moment I got through the front door back home." It was clear that Mr Howard was a flat-track playground bully, and there was a worrying and uncomfortable degree of fear within the team around him.

Whenever Mr Howard was on-call, we were using valuable time and cognitive bandwidth worrying about, and planning for, our upcoming interaction with him, a response to our level of fear (or lack of psychological safety) that may itself have affected our ability to keep patients safe. Amy Edmondson explains in *The Fearless Organization* that fear activates the brain's threat-detection centre in the amygdala, leading to fewer cognitive resources being available for processes such as analytical thinking and problem solving. "This is why it's hard for people to do their best work when they are afraid," concludes Edmondson.

One key factor determining an individual's level of psychological safety is the steepness of the hierarchical structure within their team, and their own position within that hierarchy. Medical teams in hospitals have historically been notoriously hierarchical and, although there have been recent moves to flatten the hierarchy, it remains the case that there is usually an explicit (and sometimes an implicit) rank order of seniority within our teams. New doctors, who sit right at the bottom of this pecking order, can be amongst the most vulnerable to the effects of hierarchy on psychological safety. In the next section, we will look more closely at how we can understand and respond to our position within the medical hierarchy in order to get things right.

Handling the Hierarchy

On the 28th of December 1978, United Airlines Flight 173 from JFK International Airport crashed in Portland, Oregon, resulting in the death of ten people on board. The pilot, Captain McBroom, had become overly task-focused on attempting to troubleshoot a warning light indicating that the landing gear had not successfully lowered, becoming oblivious to the growing and more serious danger of the fuel running out. However, when his colleagues in the cockpit First Officer Beebe and Flight Engineer Mendenhall belatedly became aware of the fuel issue themselves, they strongly hinted at it in their communication to Captain McBroom, but did not explicitly state the problem. In *Black Box Thinking*, Matthew Syed narrates how "the first officer and engineer could not understand why the pilot was not heading directly to the airport. . . . But he was the authority figure. He was the boss. He had the experience and the seniority. They called him 'sir'"[67]. Eight passengers and two crew members aboard United Airlines Flight 173 died that day. One of them was Flight Engineer Mendenhall. The effects of an institutional hierarchy on effective communication had cost him and nine others their lives.

The self-silencing of junior team members in healthcare can have similarly disastrous consequences. One ICU patient I was looking after with a suspected lower gastrointestinal bleed had had a normal CT angiogram, which had not identified a source of the bleeding. However, he was still needing blood transfusions to keep him stable. I wondered whether the problem might be an upper GI bleed with rapid transit time, masquerading as the bright red blood of a lower GI bleed, but subconsciously assumed that the registrar would have already considered this possibility. I said nothing, and our patient remained unwell for the next few hours. In the morning, when the consultant arrived, he made the decision for an emergency endoscopy that confirmed it was an upper GI bleed. It had been a close shave, and when the registrar and I talked about it I confessed that the possibility of an upper GI source had crossed my mind. "Well, you could have told me!" he said.

Why had I stayed silent? My registrar was approachable. We'd been working together for a while. He was a nice guy. It would have been easy to offer a suggestion. Amy Edmondson describes how a lack of psychological safety, particularly for those at the bottom of organisational hierarchies, manifests as fear of three "interpersonal risks" of appearing ignorant, incompetent or disruptive. These interpersonal risks may then prevent us from asking questions, admitting to mistakes or making suggestions respectively. "The gravitational pull of silence – even when bosses are well-meaning and don't think of themselves as intimidating – can be overwhelming," Edmondson summarises. So, is there anything we can do to help ourselves counterbalance that?

The United Airlines Flight 173 disaster was one of a series of aviation disasters in the 1970s that prompted the development of 'Crew Resource Management' (CRM) training, designed to engender more effective communication in crisis scenarios.[68] First officers, subordinate to the pilot, were taught graded assertiveness techniques, including the 'P.A.C.E.' mnemonic, which encouraged them to sequentially Probe, Alert, Challenge and declare an Emergency when attempting to escalate a safety concern. The idea was that, by beginning the interaction at a less confrontational level, crew members at a lower position in the hierarchy would be more likely to speak up. They could then make multiple, more achievable increases in assertiveness, thereby increasing the chances that the highly assertive safety-critical intervention would be made if needed. A similar tool for graded assertiveness in healthcare communication is the 'C.U.S.S.' model, in which a concern can be framed to a senior in progressively more assertive terms of being concerned, being unsure, the question being a safety issue and someone needing to stop what they are doing immediately.

The C.U.S.S. model is useful, but I think that for new doctors even the initial "I'm concerned that . . ." statement could be a difficult leap to make. After recounting an episode in which he challenged an attending surgeon who refused to change his latex gloves even as the patient on the table was going into anaphylactic shock, world-renowned patient safety expert Peter Pronovost reflected in *Safe Patients, Smart Hospitals* how difficult it could have been if he had been more junior.[69] "In this particular case, the patient was fortunate because I was already gaining a reputation and support inside Hopkins as a safety leader," he wrote. "That gave me the courage to speak up because I believed the dean and president of the hospital would most likely back me up. What if I was just starting out in my career?"

One adaptation would be to try an E-C.U.S.S. system, where 'E' is for education (Figure 3.1). In my experience, framing a patient management question as an educational issue is by far the least confrontational way to voice a concern. We can say something along the lines of, "Just for our learning, please could you tell us about why we're doing x, y and z?" Rather than starting off with challenging someone's authority even mildly, you are acknowledging that they are the expert in

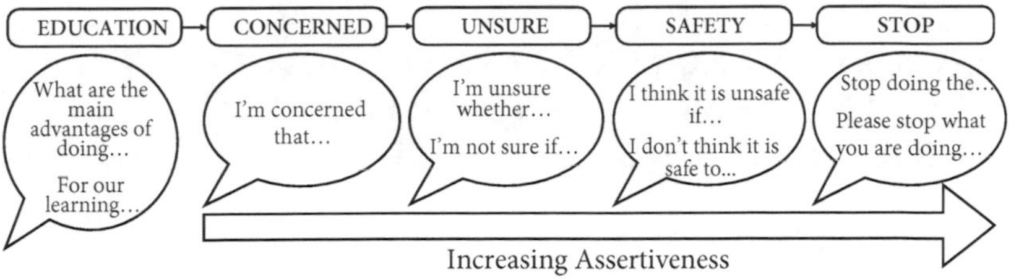
EDUCATION
CONCERNED
UNSURE
SAFETY
STOP
What are the main advantages of doing...
For our learning...
I'm concerned that...
I'm unsure whether...
I'm not sure if...
I think it is unsafe if...
I don't think it is safe to...
Stop doing the...
Please stop what you are doing...
Increasing Assertiveness

Figure 3.1 E-C.U.S.S. (Starting with an open educational question can ease a junior into discussing a concern with a senior doctor.)

the room, will have knowledge to share in this area, and that you are simply curious to know more. This strategy budgets for the most likely scenario in which the senior you are speaking to has a reason for their approach, but also leaves open the possibility to progress to the rest of the C.U.S.S. tool should the concerning or novel patient management not be explained. Crucially, the speed of progression through the E-C.U.S.S. steps must be governed by the immediacy of the possible patient safety risk. If someone is literally about to give a penicillin antibiotic to a penicillin-allergic patient, do not start with an educational question! Miss out all the other stages and tell them to stop!

A similar approach expounded by Pian-Smith and colleagues in a study conducted on Harvard anesthesiology residents is pairing advocacy and enquiry to phrase a statement that can be repeated (and perhaps strengthened if necessary) to follow a "two-challenge rule"[70]. The two-challenge rule is a communication tool borrowed from the aviation industry whereby the questioning junior will take direct action to ensure safety if an appropriate and reassuring response from their senior is not forthcoming after two consecutive challenges. Pairing advocacy and enquiry has much in common with the idea of first framing your concerns as an educational issue. In the advocacy part, the junior can begin by stating their current knowledge or understanding as relates to the issue at hand. In the enquiry part, they can ask their senior for their views or opinions on the matter (Box 3.1).

BOX 3.1 AN EXAMPLE OF PAIRED ADVOCACY AND ENQUIRY STATEMENTS, USED IN A FIRST AND SECOND CHALLENGE

1ST CHALLENGE

Advocacy: "My understanding was that left bundle branch block with chest pain can be serious . . ."
Enquiry: "What do you think about the left bundle branch block in this case?"

2ND CHALLENGE

Advocacy: "The ALS guidelines list new left bundle branch block alongside ST elevation as an indication for reperfusion . . ."
Enquiry: "Do we need to activate the cath lab pathway for this patient?"

This non-confrontational tool has the advantage that it facilitates open discussion and may offer learning opportunities regarding appropriate variations in patient management, but equally gives the junior a clear boundary for when to seek further help if their concerns are not acknowledged and addressed.

Pian-Smith's group found that teaching the advocacy-enquiry method and two-challenge rule in debriefing sessions following simulated anaesthetic scenarios increased the use of advocacy and enquiry language when challenging an attending anesthesiologist in a subsequent simulated scenario. Teaching these kinds of techniques is particularly important, since the participating residents told researchers that not being able to find the right words or phrase their question appropriately was a barrier to challenging a decision when they had a safety concern. The authors affirmed what we have seen so far in this book, writing, "clinical decisions and interventions made by trainees directly impact on the safety and wellbeing of the patients."

However, even with some useful communication tools in hand, speaking up is far from guaranteed. The difficulty is that the powerful force of self-silencing works subconsciously, sometimes completely out of reach of our conscious recognition or control. I did not go through an explicit mental process debating whether I should or shouldn't discuss my thoughts with the ICU registrar. If we have failed to recognise our self-silencing altogether, we may not get as far as employing the techniques described earlier. As with any human cognitive bias, simply learning about it and being aware of it will not be enough. We need our leaders and organisations to redesign and restructure the systems in which we work, in the knowledge and expectation that these cognitive biases will remain in play. Here, that means taking steps to permanently flatten the hierarchy.

Many consultants do recognise the dangers of a steep hierarchical structure, in which they are assumed to be correct 100% of the time and their juniors do not feel empowered to ask questions, raise concerns or (if need be) directly challenge them. Jay Jayamohan, a Consultant Paediatric Neurosurgeon at the John Radcliffe Hospital in Oxford, wrote in his memoir *Everything That Makes Us Human*,

> I give the same pep-talk to everyone who works for me. Don't trust me just because I am your boss. If you think that I'm about to do something wrong, something stupid, you shout, you stop me. I'm relying on you. And what's more, so is the patient. Even teachers make mistakes.[71]

This kind of briefing was designed to give all his team members, including theatre staff, nurses and junior doctors, a free pass to challenge their leader if they felt something was about to go wrong, safe in the knowledge that they would be thanked for speaking up.

As well as explicitly giving team members permission to challenge those at the top of the hierarchy, there are other steps some consultants take that flatten the hierarchical structure. One consultant I worked for insisted that we call her Sarah rather than "Dr Robertson". Initially I resisted, continuing with "Dr Robertson" as I had been accustomed to, believing that this was a matter of courtesy and respect; she was the consultant, after all. But she kept insisting and eventually I got the message. The offer from a consultant to call them by their first name was a simple but dramatically effective move in flattening the hierarchy. She instantly made herself more approachable for queries and concerns. Some may argue that the formal designation of "Dr so and so" is necessary to mark the status and authority of a consultant as leader of the team, separate from the other doctors and nurses who all call each other by their first names. Yet Sarah didn't need a different title to maintain her authority in the leadership position; she was a truly fantastic doctor who led by example, she was kind to her team, and we looked forward to coming to work when she was on-call. And there was no doubt about who was in charge and was taking ultimate responsibility for the patients.

Even in a psychologically safe environment where the hierarchy is somewhat flattened, it can still be difficult as the most junior doctor to get colleagues to take your concerns seriously. What can we do when we *have* made the decision to escalate a problem and are doing so loudly and clearly, but are met with a response that seems disinterested, too slow or wholly inadequate? Having discussed the issue of subconscious self-silencing when we might be right but do not speak up, we now turn to the opposite problem that occurs when we are right and are speaking up, but are struggling to be heard.

Shouting into the Wind

Halfway through a shift on a freezing January night, a new doctor called Toby was caught in the middle of an unexpected scene. He stood on a mezzanine floor in the hospital's main atrium, alongside a 24-year-old patient called Lloyd. Over the edge of the mezzanine's glass balcony was a drop stretching to the ground floor below. Lloyd was saying that he wanted to jump over it, and was beginning to make moves to do just that. "There were four doctors, and maybe five nurses, all surrounding him, all trying to reason with him not to jump into the atrium. Security were on their way to help us," Toby recounted. "He was so forthcoming, telling us what had happened in his life and why he felt that way, and from what he was saying I could understand why he would feel so sad." Before the security team arrived, Lloyd was successfully talked down, and agreed to return to the ward. The gaggle of staff dissipated, leaving Toby and Lloyd alone.

The problem was that Toby was not on a rotation in a psychiatric hospital. Lloyd was not on a psychiatric ward. Having initially come to hospital with a groin abscess, he was being cared for by the general surgery team. When Lloyd walked away from the atrium, the staff surrounding him returned to their routine work, the crisis seemingly averted. But Toby knew that more was needed. Lloyd was in a very vulnerable mental state and needed specialist care. Toby made the decision to escalate the problem, so called his boss, the surgical registrar. The registrar was kind, but this was not something surgeons were used to dealing with, so he suggested calling the nurse site manager. "I called the site manager, explained that Lloyd was expressing these suicidal thoughts, and said that I didn't think it was safe for him to be on this surgical ward," Toby explained.

> It wasn't a safe environment. The nurses were very short-staffed and they couldn't provide one-to-one care. They were in and out checking on Lloyd but they couldn't be there all the time. I explained explicitly to the site manager that he was a danger to himself. I tried everything to escalate it but nobody was listening. Our ward sister tried to escalate as well but nobody was listening to her either.

Toby was sitting at the ward desk, getting nowhere. He had escalated within his team. He had escalated outside of his team. As he sat listening to the rings, waiting for the operator to connect yet another phone call for him to explain the situation, the crash buzzer erupted. It was coming from Lloyd's room. As he entered, followed by the ward nurses, Toby looked in absolute horror at what he saw. Using strips torn from his bedsheet tied together and then to the curtain rail, Lloyd had hung himself.

Toby sprang into action, lifting Lloyd as high as he could whilst one of the nurses grabbed the scissors from the resuscitation trolley and frantically cut him down. His body was still and lifeless, not moving and not breathing. Toby supported Lloyd's neck and managed his airway as the nurses started CPR. Soon, amazingly, his pulse returned. The crash team arrived, intubated him and took him to the ICU. It was a couple of days later that Toby and his colleagues found out that Lloyd had survived. "I went to see him on the ICU," Toby recalled. "He was awake and talking, and regretful, saying that he wished he hadn't done it, and thanking us for being there for him."

The incident has stayed with Toby, and always will. I was struck by the terrifying image of your worst fears for a patient being realised in such violent and distressing circumstances, despite your best efforts to prevent it. What toll might that have taken? Yet Toby has gone on to become one of the most motivated and impressive surgical trainees I know. Although Lloyd's acute suicidality is a particularly harrowing example, there are many such instances where our course of action in escalating concerns is safety-critical. In this case, Toby's efforts were overtaken by the speed of events, and he was hampered by the lack of a clear system for ward doctors to escalate psychiatric issues in a general hospital, but there is still much to learn from the sensible way he approached the struggle to be heard.

Firstly, Toby immediately skipped to the "safety" section of the C.U.S.S. tool, using an appropriate level of assertiveness for the situation he was faced with. He explicitly stated to his seniors that Lloyd could not be kept safe in his current ward environment. When I asked him about it, Toby had done this naturally without any prior knowledge of the C.U.S.S. strategy, but by teaching different communication tools we can give new doctors confidence that they are responding reasonably and professionally to the situation in front of them. Toby had also been extremely quick to set about getting the help he needed and had enlisted the help of the senior nurse on the ward.

When discussing the chain of command for managing uncertainty in Chapter 1, we saw how senior doctors such as registrars and consultants may seek help from another specialty when they do not know how best to proceed. Once a problem has been passed up the chain within a team, help from another team is often sought. This process is referral, where a problem has already been escalated to some degree but is best solved with input of knowledge or skills from a different team. Even if the task of referring is handed back down the chain to the junior members to do it on the senior's behalf, it is still the same mechanism. When Toby's registrar was also unsure how to get the required help, he suggested calling the Nurse Site Manager, the most senior nurse in the hospital, which Toby then did.

However, new doctors should also be empowered to call directly on alternative sources of help if the situation necessitates it, particularly if they are not getting a timely response, an adequate response or any response at all from their immediate seniors. This can be thought of as 'sideways escalation' (Figure 3.2). In the vast majority of cases sideways escalation should not be necessary, and it is usually preferable for issues to be escalated 'vertically' in the usual fashion, even using an 'over-bleep' if required. Yet new doctors should feel confident to think flexibly, seek alternative help and escalate sideways if the situation demands it. Sideways escalation should not be misused as a route to an apparently easier phone call to a registrar thought more likely to be helpful. After all, that would suggest a problem with the approachability or civility of the first registrar. Sideways escalation should be reserved for when it is really needed.

The final important learning points from Toby's story are to be found in the exemplary way the ward team handled the crisis when

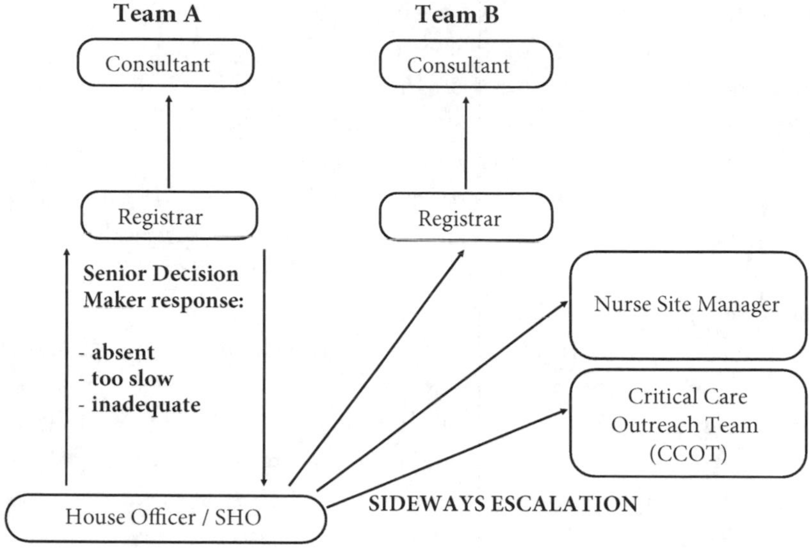

Figure 3.2 Sideways escalation is the seeking of help from outside your own team when traditional 'vertical' escalation has failed. Possible sources of help might include a different team's registrar, the Nurse Site Manager or the Critical Care Outreach Team (CCOT).

they found Lloyd. The team worked and managed to perform in an immensely pressurised scenario. In this chapter's discussion of how new doctors can get things right, we have come full circle back to emergencies. We will conclude with learning some more about performance-enhancing mental strategies that can help us get things right when managing an extremely sick, acutely unwell patient.

Beat The Stress, Fool!

At the end of Chapter 1 we saw how our levels of stress can affect performance, which was placed within the broader discussion of how new doctors think and make decisions. We focused in particular on the idea of 'cognitive appraisal' of a stressful situation, which is our perception

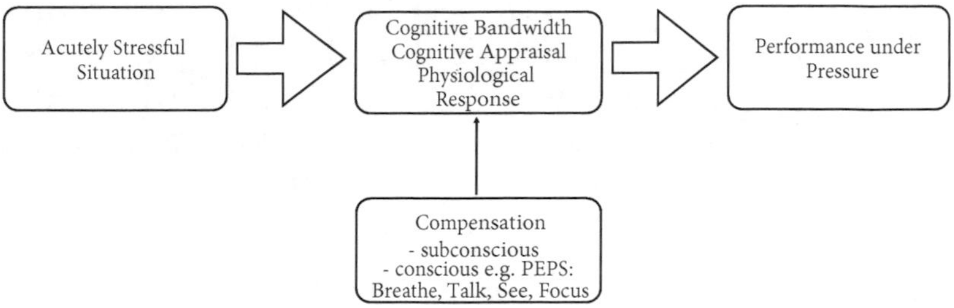

Figure 3.3 Cognitive bandwidth, cognitive appraisal and the physiological stress response help determine our performance under pressure. Both subconscious and consciously deployed compensatory mechanisms come to our aid in times of acute stress. PEPS are Performance-Enhancing Psychological Skills.

of the scenario, its riskiness and what the possible outcomes might mean for us personally. Cognitive appraisal sits alongside cognitive bandwidth (something inversely related to our level of mental overload) and our physiological response to stress in determining whether or not we perform as required when under pressure (Figure 3.3). We saw in Chapter 1 how a negative cognitive appraisal, where we perceive that our coping mechanisms might be overwhelmed, is linked with impaired performance, and considered how new doctors will begin to make more positive cognitive appraisals as they build clinical experience. However, in the heat of the moment some more immediate tactics are needed.

In 2017, Michael Lauria and colleagues wrote a paper in *Annals of Emergency Medicine* describing four performance-enhancing psychological skills (PEPS) that have the potential to increase new doctors' cognitive bandwidth, increase their perceived coping ability leading to more positive cognitive appraisals of situations and moderate the physiological response to stress.[72] These four PEPS are related to Breathing, Talking (self-talk), Seeing (mental visualisation) and Focusing, with BTSF spelling out the mnemonic "Beat The Stress, Fool!" For new doctors, spending time learning about and practising psychological skills may not seem relevant to their work, and the language of crew resource management and "PEPS" may seem best kept for anaesthetists, intensivists and emergency physicians in the resuscitation room, where it was developed. But here we should return to the concept of cognitive appraisal. It is how a situation *feels* to us that matters. It may be that the psychological challenges facing two new doctors dealing with a seizing and unconscious patient on the ward for the first time have more in common with those experienced by an ICU registrar dealing with a difficult airway in a polytrauma patient than it would first appear. We must each rise to our own level of challenge.

The breathing component of BTSF is to use a technique called 'square breathing' or 'tactical breathing' when we feel our anxiety levels rise in the face of a stressful scenario. This involves taking a deep, slow breath in for 4 seconds, holding it for 4 seconds, breathing out slowly for 4 seconds, and then holding our lungs empty for 4 seconds, imagining the equal four sides of a square as we go. The exact duration of each step isn't important, but doing the breathing *slowly* is; the aim is to bring our rising respiratory rate and heart rate under control first of all, creating the conditions in which our runaway thought processes can follow suit. Hearing about square breathing reminded me of *The House of God* and the Fat Man's third law stating, "At a cardiac arrest the first procedure is to take your own pulse"[73]. Square breathing doesn't have to be a big deal and doesn't need to be regularly practised each day. It could just be something to try briefly for half a minute when you are next faced with a situation that represents an acutely stressful challenge.

The next part (T) is about self-talk. When we chatted about the difficulties of starting work as a new doctor, Sanith remarked, "When you know you've got all this work that you need to get through, you're also battling your own sense of self-efficacy, of how good you are. Feeling rubbish and like you can't do something can really affect your confidence." Lauria and colleagues explain that self-efficacy is "an individual's perception that he or she can successfully perform a task" and that this can be boosted by positive self-talk. The broad human negativity bias, of which loss aversion is one part, gives rise to a ratio for positive to negative feedback that has been proposed to be around 3:1, whereby we need three positive pieces of feedback just to balance out a single negative one.[74] I suspect the same goes for self-talk.

When we are wracked with doubts about our own abilities in frightening and acutely stressful situations, it is imperative to fight back with positive self-talk. We need to actively tell ourselves that we can do this. Professor Sara Gray, an emergency medicine and critical care specialist at the University of Toronto, describes the importance of positive self-talk as follows: "If you can work together with your inner voice . . . there's evidence to show that you can resuscitate better, or have better bedside performance, if you're not wasting all your cognitive processing power fighting with the voice in your head"[75]. We need to be kind to ourselves and consciously practise positive self-talk to develop an inner voice that, with time, can become our closest ally in times of great stress.

The 'S' in the mnemonic is for seeing, meaning the use of mental practice in the mind's eye to run through the steps of a practical procedure or the management of a medical emergency before it actually happens. This technique is well-established in the field of sports psychology. We are used to hearing about how Olympic athletes work with their psychologists to visualise the perfect 100m sprint, triple jump or javelin throw. They understand that visualising things going right increases the odds that it will play out that way in reality. Although the exact mechanism by which mental practice improves performance is not yet known, imaging studies have revealed clear neural correlates suggesting that simply imagining and visualising the steps in a performance or procedure activates the same regions of the brain and neural networks as actually doing that task.[76]

Researchers are now shining a light on how mental practice can be put to use for clinicians who need to perform under pressure.

A small, randomised controlled study of 20 novice surgeons found that 30 minutes of mental practice before each Virtual Reality laparoscopic cholecystectomy undertaken significantly improved performance compared with a control group who received an online lecture.[77] Another randomised study showed that "Surgical Cognitive Simulation" improved trainees' real-world performance on a surgical curriculum programme assessment four months later.[78] For new doctors, the same benefits are likely to be accrued for mental practice of ward-based procedures, but mental pre-rehearsal can also be a powerful tool for preparing yourself to deal with emergencies. Although the early management of a medical emergency is different from executing the motor tasks needed for a procedure, the algorithmic approach still lends itself well to mental practice. Cardiac arrest: call for help, 2222, start CPR, defibrillator pads on, pause compressions, rhythm check, shock if required, continue CPR. Anaphylaxis: call for help, 2222, remove the source, 500 micrograms of adrenaline IM, high-flow oxygen, IV access, bolus crystalloid. For the most high-pressure scenarios we could find ourselves in, especially those which are either very rare or in which we are inexperienced, we can mentally run through the key actions. Peter Brindley, a Professor of Critical Care Medicine in Alberta, Canada, phrased it simply: "The best simulator in the world is the human brain"[79].

Finally, the 'F' in "Beat The Stress, Fool!" is for Focus. Lauria and his colleagues suggest that we should choose a "trigger word" to signal to ourselves that we are entering a difficult phase of work under stress where total attention is required. We might whisper "Focus!" under our breath as we begin to help an extremely unwell patient. "The ability to hone one's attention and focus on important clinical tasks during emergencies is crucial," Lauria writes. Although the evidence base for this last of Lauria's four PEPS comes from fields outside of medicine, the authors argue that this simple technique should be usable in any high-stress environment. I'm going to give it a try.

Over the course of this chapter, we have considered some of the elements of complex health systems, at the institutional, team and individual levels, which are important in allowing new doctors to get things right. Although there are deep-rooted cognitive biases that make it against our nature to focus on and learn about the factors that help things to go right, we have seen in detail the possible effects of civility, psychological safety, a flattened hierarchy and performance-enhancing psychological skills on the safety of our patients. These pieces are no substitute for extensive knowledge, training and clinical acumen, but they are hidden facilitators that need to be acknowledged both by new doctors and the leaders of the systems they work in.

In Chapter 4, we turn our attention to one of the toughest parts of any new doctor's work – the night shift. With fewer staff, and fewer senior staff, present in the hospital at night, new doctors play a more vital role. The darkness of the night brings all of the issues we have discussed so far into sharp relief. We will look at the risks associated with working at night and explore how we can see clearly, and think clearly, in the night.

"No man knows till he has suffered from the night how sweet and dear to his heart and eye the morning can be."

Bram Stoker, *Dracula*

4

NIGHT MODE

HOW CAN WE KEEP PATIENTS SAFE AT NIGHT?

The Hospital at Night

The hospital is a different place at night. Your footsteps ring out against empty corridors, which only a few hours ago were bustling with elderly people being pushed in wheelchairs, families visiting their relatives' wards, hospital charity volunteers recruiting for the fun run and patients being transported to CT scans with their entourage of beeping monitors, equipment, nurses and doctors. Now the commotion and hullabaloo of the daytime are gone, the humdrum and routine comings and goings of hospital life finished for another day. Left behind are only the skeleton crew of staff deemed necessary to cope with the emergent and the urgent, the patients and the medicine that cannot wait until the sun rises and the hospital machine boots up once again.

At night, with the monotony of discharge summaries, routine blood tests and referral letters stripped away, junior doctors are cast as night watchmen to keep the patients safe until morning, and our contribution suddenly feels more vital, more necessary and more valuable than it ever did in the day.

With fewer staff, and fewer senior staff, in the hospital at night, the level of responsibility shouldered by new doctors is categorically different from the daytime. Almost by definition, the patients we are seeing are sicker than our daytime patients would be, and there is potential for a frightening volume problem to arise if the number of new admissions or inpatient deteriorations on a particular night overwhelms hospital staff. Furthermore, our task sorting, prioritisation and execution has to occur whilst fighting against accumulating fatigue and an internal body clock that is befuddled as to why we're not safely tucked up at home asleep. It is the equivalent of requiring the spinning plates act discussed in Chapter 1 to be performed with one eye shut, slightly drunk, standing on a balance beam. The patients being acutely unwell, the lower levels of staffing and the profoundly non-physiological demands placed on our bodies and brains mean that the time when most is required of us is also the time when we are cognitively at our most vulnerable.

When I moved to the Small Hospital for the second rotation of my first year, I was rostered to start on night shifts straight away, which was a daunting prospect. Just before leaving the DGH, I got some advice from one of the experienced SHOs on our ward. "Well, it's a ward cover role at night," he told me. "Your job is literally just to keep everyone alive until the morning." I must have looked perturbed, since he followed that up by saying, "I'm only half-joking – at night you just need to prioritise and focus on the urgent issues, the things that can't wait." I soon learnt that he was correct. There was no slack in the system, winter had set in, and we were extremely busy. During out-of-hours working, which includes evenings and weekends as well as nights, hospitals generally operate on what is known as 'minimum safe staffing', supplying each department with just enough doctors and nurses to get by. It is worth considering that Monday to Friday 8 am to 5 pm accounts for only 45 of the 168 hours in each week, which is just 27% of the time. We tend to think of daytime staffing levels as the norm, and out-of-hours staffing as the exception, but this is an illusion. Although scheduled procedures and most key treatment decisions take place in weekday daylight hours, the immediate responsibility for a patient's care should they deteriorate will fall to an out-of-hours team 73% of the time. So, are the patients less safe out-of-hours? And specifically, are they less safe at night?

Safety in the Dark

In 2010, Maggs and Mallet retrospectively analysed a year's worth of emergency admissions to a medium-sized DGH, finding that mortality was significantly higher for patients admitted out-of-hours compared with in-hours, and for those admitted at night compared with during the daytime.[80] Crucially though, they only adjusted their data for age and sex, not for admission diagnosis or underlying co-morbidities, acknowledging therefore that it was not clear to what extent the mortality differences were due to the patients admitted out-of-hours or overnight just being sicker to start off with. However, they did comment that the fact the differences were still seen in late mortality (deaths occurring at >7 days since admission) as well as in overall mortality (all deaths) suggested a strong role for patient factors at admission. Any variations in healthcare quality arising around the time of admission would be expected to have a much smaller effect on the deaths that occurred more than seven days down the line. Just as we saw at the start of the book with the questions surrounding Black Wednesday mortality and new doctors' supposed collective incompetence, it is an obvious but understated truth that patient factors probably matter at least as much as in-hospital factors in determining outcomes.

Given the confounding factor of night admission patients, as a group, possibly being sicker than the daytime admission cohort, and the difficulty of disentangling pre-hospital and patient factors from the care someone receives in hospital, mortality rates are too much of a blunt instrument to analyse safety at night. We need to consider the effect of the night for the prioritisation, assessment and decision-making affecting any patient who deteriorates. At the level of the individual, the question is whether becoming unwell at 3 am means you will be less safe than a similar patient *who became equally unwell* at 3 pm the preceding afternoon. Do the effects of night shift working and accumulating fatigue on healthcare workers produce unwanted variation in the clinical assessment and management of comparable day and night patients?

In a 2018 report titled "Fatigue and Sleep Deprivation – The Impact of Different Working Patterns on Doctors", the British Medical Association highlighted the negative cognitive and psychomotor effects of fatigue and sleep deprivation on task performance, working memory capacity and attention.[81] Whilst their review did comment that the available evidence was limited, they pointed to multiple observational studies that linked self-reported, fatigue-related medical errors to patient injury or mortality. They also highlighted a prospective randomised study that compared rates of serious medical errors made by critical care interns in the United States working shifts longer than 24 hours versus shifts of less than 16 hours.[82] Unsurprisingly, interns on the rota that included traditional 'extended duration shifts' lasting over 24 hours committed 36% more serious medical errors, 21% more medication errors and 5.6 times as many serious diagnostic errors. Although these findings from the US are not directly generalisable worldwide, since their residency shifts are often dramatically longer than those in comparable health systems, the key message is clear – accumulating fatigue is likely to decrease the safety of those in our care.

The traditional American-style 'extended duration' shift seems far too long to be optimal for patient safety, but how long is too long? And when exactly should we be most alert to the clinical dangers of mounting fatigue? In a non-systematic review article titled "Shift work, safety and productivity" published in *Occupational Medicine* in 2003, Folkard and Tucker combined data from three studies into shift duration and accident risk and found that the risk of accidents after 12 hours worked was approximately double that seen at 8 hours worked.[83] Risk was relatively constant in the first 8 hours of a shift, but then seemed to increase dramatically. They also showed a similar increase in risk across four successive night shifts, supporting the anecdotal feeling of most doctors that, by the fourth night in a row, you are approaching your limit for retaining an acceptable level of performance. We will separately consider the sleep physiology that determines the riskiest period within a given night shift later in the chapter.

Many new doctors told me stories of mistakes they have made whilst tired on night shifts. Jessie, a first-year doctor, recounted clerking new admissions onto the vascular ward one night, which involved prescribing the patients' regular medications. A 73-year-old gentleman called Henry Morrison took Bed 2a, while 75-year-old Harry Morris occupied the adjacent Bed 2b. Somewhere amongst the flurry of papers in the doctors' office in the early hours, Jessie confused the two patients' records and prescribed Harry's medications on Henry's chart, and vice versa. Fortunately, the error was uncovered at the morning meds round when their nurse checked her printed handover sheet and said, "Henry, you're not diabetic are you? You seem to have been prescribed quite a large dose of insulin." It was a very near miss.

Colin, one of Jessie's colleagues in her cohort, also had a near miss with a prescription error at night. When admitting Mr Patel, a 52-year-old lawyer, to the Acute Medical Unit (AMU) with a swollen, red and painful right calf, he was lulled into a false sense of security by this seemingly simple case of possible deep vein thrombosis requiring a treatment dose of low molecular weight heparin. Colin took Mr Patel's medical history, examined the leg and prescribed the necessary blood thinner. "It was about 3 am on the third of four nights," Colin remembered. "I was more or less functioning on auto-pilot." Colin's diagnosis and plan wasn't incorrect per se, but the problem was that the ED SHO had already given Mr Patel the blood thinner. It was prescribed on the back of the separate ED chart, which the tired Colin had forgotten to check. When the nurse approached Mr Patel with the blood thinning injection, he exclaimed "Haven't I already had that one?" The fact that Mr Patel was an engaged patient who had understood his treatment plan came to Colin's aid. "I was lucky it wasn't a patient who was confused or had dementia," Colin reflected.

The possible effects of fatigue on medical error rates are concerning, yet more concerning still is the fact that we may not recognise when we are becoming most hazardous for our patients. Van Dongen and colleagues in 2003 compared psychomotor vigilance test (PVT) performance across 14 days in groups of subjects that were allowed either 8, 6 or 4 hours of sleep per night, as well as in a group undergoing total sleep restriction for three days.[84] They also collected Stanford Sleepiness Scale self-ratings from the participants. Crucially, even as PVT lapses increased over the 14 days in the 6 hours and 4 hours sleep-restricted groups relative to the 8 hours per night controls, the subjective sleepiness scores levelled off. The subjects were unaware of the effect the cumulative sleep restriction was having on their performance.

In a similar way that the Dunning–Kruger bias we encountered in Chapter 1 produces unconscious incompetence where we don't know what we don't know, these data suggest that tired doctors accumulating sleep debt over a series of night shifts will be poor judges of their own fatigue. They will therefore be less likely to do anything about it. With the caveat that PVT performance – pressing a button quickly in response to a stimulus – is not the same thing as safe doctoring, it is reasonable to question whether the effects of fatigue on clinically vital higher cognitive functions such as complex reasoning and decision-making might go similarly unrecognised. We may be, almost literally, sleepwalking into a state of impaired performance, resulting in increased risk for our patients. Against this backdrop of compromised cognitive abilities, lower staffing levels mean that doctors on the nightshift face a higher burden of choices than they ordinarily would in the daytime. In the coming sections we will look more closely at how increasing mental fatigue affects how doctors think and decide.

In Shock

Gwen Jones was an elderly woman who lived in a small cottage on the edge of the town park, around a mile and a half from the university where she had worked as a research assistant in the biochemistry labs until her retirement nearly 20 years ago. She had lived alone for the past five years since her husband Ted had died, filling her weekly schedule with coffee mornings, outdoor aerobics in the park, visits from her grandchildren and her work as treasurer for the amateur dramatic society. It was good to keep busy. It held back the loneliness after Ted had gone, a feeling that despite the passing years never truly went away.

She was in quite good health for a woman in her 80s but did have an irregular heartbeat her GP had called 'Atrial Fibrillation'. It meant she had to have a blood thinner to reduce her risk of strokes, but that wasn't so bad. Lots of her friends had much worse to cope with. She used to take a tablet called Warfarin, which was a nuisance because the dose kept changing according to her INR blood tests, which were far too frequent for her liking. A couple of years ago, however, they had switched her to a new blood thinner called Apixaban, which was much simpler – you just took the same tablet twice per day. She also took a statin, something for the blood pressure, and some ibuprofen now and again for her left knee. Occasionally, she pushed her luck with her knee and the aerobics, but no matter. All in all, life wasn't so bad.

One Thursday afternoon in January, though, Gwen noticed some abdominal pain and when she opened her bowels, she found that the stool was very dark, almost black. It was all very strange. Her knee had been playing up that week as usual, but she'd never had anything like this before. She put it to the back of her mind and went back to watching TV. However, around 10 pm after dinner the same thing happened again. Her stool was black, and she was feeling rather sick and dizzy. Gwen didn't like to trouble anyone but gave her daughter Mandy a call. Mandy was worried, insisted on coming over right away, and when she saw how pale Gwen looked she decided to call 999. It was a good decision, but unfortunately this was the last good decision Gwen experienced for the next several hours.

In the Emergency Department, it was pandemonium. There had been 156 patients in the department when the night team had come on shift at 9 pm, and the building had been designed for 40. There were patients on trolleys in every available space, staff rushing here and there, and ambulance crews queued up outside trying to hand over their patients. The doctors and nurses were exhausted, and they didn't feel like they were making any progress. They tried to work out who was the sickest, who needed to be seen first. Meanwhile, more and more patients kept on arriving. In amongst the chaos, Gwen was briefly seen by a new doctor sometime after 1 am, her history taken, her blood tests checked and a referral made to the AMU for rectal bleeding. She waited in the queue for a bed.

At 3.45 am, Gwen was wheeled into the AMU and transferred to a bed, where the nurses tried to take her observations at admission. She had a heart rate of 155 beats per minute, but the blood pressure cuff wouldn't read a number. Gwen's hands were stone cold and she was deathly pale. Laura, the medical SHO, stopped what she was doing and got to work. She scanned through the ED note on the computer: "Rectal bleeding . . . dark stools . . . Haemoglobin 60 g/L . . . Urea 23 mmol/L . . . Plan, discussed with ED consultant, admit to medicine for PR bleeding." What treatment had she had so far? Very little, it seemed. It looked like the team in the ED had decided upon precisely nothing. Why hadn't they acted? And how had a consultant signed off on this glaring omission? Laura was in shock. But for the moment, that wasn't the priority. Gwen was in haemorrhagic shock and looked to be peri-arrest.

"Katie, come and help me, there's a big bleed!" Laura said, summoning the other SHO on the unit, who she had known since the start of medical school. Next, she hit 2222 on the phone at the desk saying "Major Haemorrhage Protocol, Acute Medical Unit, Bay 1." The two SHOs drew on every ounce of their experience, managing to get a large cannula into Gwen's left arm, ready for the arriving O negative blood transfusion. Gwen didn't even flinch as the drip was inserted, drifting in and out of consciousness as she teetered on the brink of cardiovascular collapse. Within minutes, the crash team arrived to help stabilise Gwen, while Katie called the haematologists and arranged access to Prothrombin Complex Concentrate to help reverse Gwen's Apixaban. The on-call pharmacist delivered it. The senior sister prepared it. The anaesthetics registrar booked the emergency theatre ready for an endoscopy that would prove life saving for Gwen. The gastroenterology registrar and his consultant were already en-route to the hospital, responding to the call of the hospital-issue mobile phones that stayed by their pillows all night. At 5.30 am, the endoscopy revealed a bleeding stomach ulcer, which was fixed with clips and adrenaline. Gwen recovered slowly on the ward over the next six days. The well-oiled emergency team had functioned perfectly, and disaster was averted.

Fatigued Doctors and Decision Fatigue

In their omission to act upon Gwen's blood test results or take any steps to treat her deteriorating condition, one factor affecting the over-stretched ED team is likely to have been 'decision fatigue'. This term was coined by social psychologist Roy F Baumeister for the way in which making a high volume of decisions causes a decrease in decision quality.[85] Like many scientific discoveries, the decision fatigue effect was stumbled upon serendipitously. Baumeister's research group had already demonstrated that willpower was a finite resource that could be depleted, showing for example that participants forced to resist eating candy would subsequently be less able to resist a plate of cookies, or that subjects who expended willpower refraining from showing emotion watching a sad movie would then perform worse on a test of grip strength duration, used as a proxy measure for willpower. However, it was only when postdoctoral fellow Jean Twenge realised that she felt the same kind of mental exhaustion after an intense weekend of wedding planning, which had involved serial decision-making, that the group investigated the effects of deciding.

Twenge's hunch was correct. Experiments showed that forcing people to make lots of decisions in a row reduced their willpower. And crucially, depleted willpower has a knock-on effect on how the brain deals with subsequent decisions. "No matter how rational and high-minded you try to be, you can't make decision after decision without paying a biological price," wrote John Tierney in a *New York Times* essay adapted from a book he co-authored with Baumeister on the subject.[86] "The more choices you make throughout the day, the harder each one becomes for your brain, and eventually it looks for shortcuts." On the night shift, the reduced doctor to patient ratio exacerbates the problem, producing a particularly high burden of decisions and triggering the subconscious use of shortcuts.

The shortcuts underlying decision fatigue's impact on decision quality can take a number of possible forms (Figure 4.1). Firstly, decision fatigue may cause us to become more reckless and impulsive, leading to increased use of heuristics, those clinical experience-dependent mental shortcuts that allow us to think fast and quickly reach a judgement. When our decision-making becomes less slow and deliberate in this way, and we rely on these leaps of faith in our clinical reasoning, we benefit from their speed and efficiency but incur the potentially heavy cost of decreased accuracy and safety.

The second possible effect of decision fatigue is that we take the ultimate energy-conserving shortcut and do nothing – we procrastinate on the decision-making task. At first glance this certainly seems like a negative effect, but is it necessarily a bad thing for patient safety? In

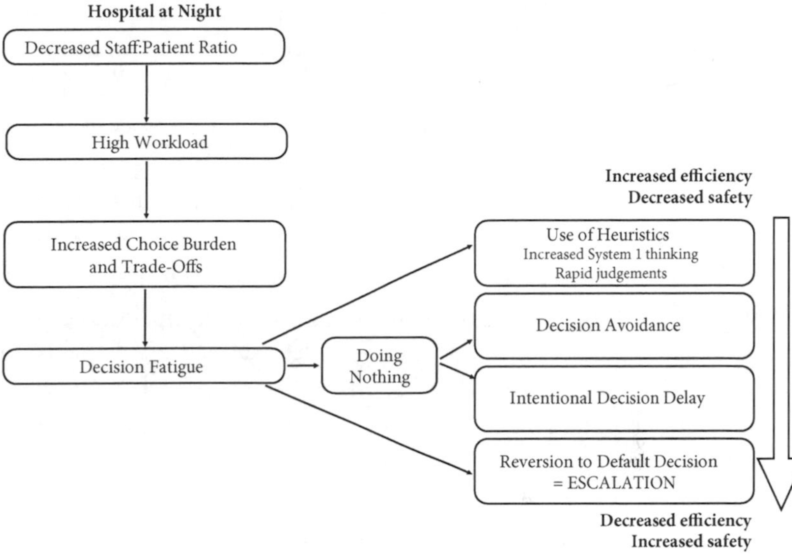

Figure 4.1 Decision fatigue at night. Staffing conditions in the hospital at night increase the likelihood of decision fatigue, which has a range of possible consequences.

our discussion of multi-tasking in Chapter 1, I suggested that there is intentional and unintentional task switching, which would be helpful and unhelpful respectively. Similarly, the merits of procrastinating on a decision depend on whether we are doing this consciously and deliberately, or subconsciously and without realising it. If we have enough mental resources to slowly evaluate a problem and we conclude that it can safely be left for the consultant on the morning ward round, that is intentional decision delay. Of course, we have still made a decision (the decision to leave it for now and hand it over), but we have deferred writing or not writing that prescription, ordering or not ordering that scan. If, on the other hand, accumulating decision fatigue goes unrecognised and makes us fail to address a decision altogether, we have become decision avoidant.

One example that occurs overnight is the sometimes-tricky decision on whether a new patient should have venous thromboembolism (VTE) prophylaxis prescribed. If they have risk factors for developing blood clots (which most inpatients do) but unclear or uncertain risk factors for bleeding, what is the best thing to do? At 4.30 am on the third of four nights, we are not the best people to make this decision. Actually, there is no need for us to decide right now, since the first dose wouldn't be due until 6 pm in the evening. We can hand the task over to the morning team. We can intentionally delay the decision. Conversely, if the strain of the night's choices causes the VTE decision to slip from our focus, such that we neither decide nor hand it over, decision fatigue has become dangerous, and the patient's safety now depends on someone else catching the error.

A third kind of shortcut that occurs in response to decision fatigue is that we become more likely to select the default option. In other words, when the brain has made too many decisions, it opts for the easiest option, the path of least resistance. In 2019, Allan and colleagues published an analysis of the triage decisions made by nurses working for the NHS Scotland 'NHS 24' telephone helpline, a service designed to assess callers' symptoms and advise them on whether or not they should see a healthcare professional, and with what degree of urgency.[87] The study included 150 nurses' work over two full shifts, a sample amounting to approximately 4000 phone calls, and evaluated whether either an increasing length of time or a higher number of calls taken since a nurse's last break affected their odds of making the default conservative decision to refer the patient urgently to either primary or secondary care.

The results showed that for every additional call since the most recent break (or the start of the shift if no break had yet been taken), the odds of a conservative decision increased by 5.5%. For every additional hour worked since the most recent break, the odds increased by 20.5%. Crucially, there was no effect of total number of calls taken in the shift, or of total time worked, and decision-making was restored to baseline after a break. It seems that it was the number of consecutive decisions taken without a break, without an opportunity to restore cognitive resources, which was driving decision fatigue and resulting in a more conservative tendency to refer a patient in for further assessment. In this clinical context, the default option of referring the patient was a safe one, allowing the patient to be seen in-person by another healthcare professional. The system offered a natural fail-safe for the effects of decision fatigue.

However, any safety-enhancing effects of a shift towards the default decision, akin to a 'status-quo bias' taking hold, will depend on each individual's mindset and the default choices available to them within a given situation, organisation and departmental culture. For new doctors in their early months and years of practice, it is essential that the easiest option available to them is to escalate their concerns. Their default option has to be to bump problems up the chain. Getting help needs to be the path of least resistance. And although the duty of the new doctor is to treat escalation as their default, the lessons from Chapter 3 tell us that senior doctors need to be available and approachable for this to remain the case. The moment juniors become hesitant to discuss issues for fear of rudeness, reproach or humiliation, the dial swings towards more dangerous defaults.

Aside from the decision volume problem on any on-call shift, there is a deeper, more pervasive reason why over-stretched doctors become vulnerable to decision fatigue. It has to do with the effect of trade-offs. In 2010, a research team led by economist Dean Spears of Princeton University asked residents of either richer or poorer villages around Rajasthan in India to choose whether or not to buy some soap, which was offered at a healthy discount of 60% off the retail price. The residents were then given the classic handgrip duration test of willpower mentioned earlier. Startlingly, in the poorer villages, where the choice of whether or not to buy the soap represented an economic trade-off even with the 60% discount, willpower on the subsequent handgrip task was significantly lower than in the richer villages.[88]

In an accompanying control condition where the handgrip task was done *before* the soap purchase decision was presented, there was no significant difference. Decision-making requiring trade-offs reduces our willpower, and therefore may quicken the onset of decision fatigue.

When looking after multiple patients, often spread out across several different wards, doctors at night and out-of-hours must constantly make trade-off triage decisions regarding which patient to see first. During my nights covering the surgical wards as a first-year doctor I remember needing to decide between a 68-year-old woman with new fevers, abdominal pain and a falling blood pressure; a 40-year-old man passing frank blood into his catheter bag on the urology ward; an unwell child with appendicitis needing antibiotics on the other side of the hospital; as well as Pablo, an elderly Spanish man who was dying and whose family wanted to understand what was happening to him. Who was the sickest? Whose needs were the most pressing? We make triage-based trade-offs before we have even started addressing the patients' issues, which often then present risk-benefit clinical decisions that are trade-offs in their own right. The sheer number of decisions that have to be made, combined with the fact that a significant proportion of them represent trade-offs, means that eventually our brains gravitate towards quality-reducing shortcuts. Overall, the potential impacts of decision fatigue are significant. But is there anything we can actually do about it?

Fighting Decision Fatigue

Fortunately, researchers have identified a number of ways we can reduce, though not fully eliminate, the effects of decision fatigue. First of all, we can try to just decide less. President Barack Obama was well aware of the problem of decision fatigue. "You'll see I only wear blue or grey suits," he explained to *Vanity Fair* magazine in 2012.[89] "I'm trying to pare down decisions. I don't want to make decisions about what I'm eating or what I'm wearing, because I have too many other decisions to make." He understood that our mental decision-making resources are finite and will be depleted even by making choices about the small stuff. Of course, it is much easier to follow this strategy if the White House chef prepares all your meals and your mode of transport is always The Beast, Marine One or Air Force One, but there are good principles here for us all. We should pre-decide what we'll eat on night shifts. We should pre-plan what time to wake up and how we'll get to and from the hospital. And it's another great reason to just wear scrubs.

This may all seem slightly over the top, but limiting the decisions we make in the non-important areas of our lives around a set of night shifts is a key way to reduce the potential impact of decision fatigue, and something that many doctors are already doing. "I try and sort out the rest of my life beforehand, so that I only have to worry about the night shifts," my friend Ben told me. "I buy food that I like in advance and get it all ready. It's important to recognise that you shouldn't try to do anything around the night shifts – that's when things start to go very wrong." Perhaps he might have added that you also shouldn't try to *decide* anything around the night shifts. In *The Paradox of Choice*, Barry Schwartz puts it this way:

> by using rules, presumptions, standards, and routines to constrain ourselves and limit the decisions we face, we can make life more manageable, which gives us more time to devote ourselves to other people and to the decisions that we can't or don't want to avoid.[90]

This thinking applies perfectly to doctors working at night. With the inherent difficulties of the night shift, we should be making decisions about one thing and one thing only – our patients.

Another important step is to make taking breaks a priority, and to promote a group culture where breaks are encouraged as an essential part of maintaining safe performance. As we saw in the Allan study, taking a break had the power to reset decision-making to baseline, winding the clock back on decision fatigue even when the total time on shift was only getting longer. Yet guaranteeing consistent and appropriate rest periods with enough colleagues to cover the proper number of breaks is easier said than done. Furthermore, when workloads are seriously high it is easy to feel that stopping for any length of time will only make the situation worse, that you cannot afford to spend time eating, drinking or relaxing when there are more and more issues that need addressing. Almost always, the gain in efficiency and restored decision-making ability obtained from a break will more than pay back the time spent taking it. However, on the occasions where there are multiple, truly unwell patients to deal with at once, it can be the case that a whole 20 minutes sat down doing nothing is out of the question. Enter the 'micro-break'.

Micro-breaks are short breaks lasting anything from 90 seconds to 5 minutes, which have been shown to go some way towards alleviating the decline in cognitive performance associated with continuous time on task.[91] In 2017, Park and colleagues performed a multicentre cohort study of 66 surgeons investigating the effects of "targeted stretching micro-breaks" (TSMBs) on surgeons' self-reported pain scores and their perceptions of their own physical and mental operative performance.[92] The cohort completed 193 procedures on the standard day and 148 procedures on the TSMBs day, but crucially there was no significant difference in procedure duration. Even though the surgeons stopped on occasion for a micro-break, this didn't cause their procedures to take any longer, backing up the idea that breaks pay back the time costs they incur. Furthermore, the surgeons perceived increases in their physical and mental focus of 57% and 38% respectively from taking TSMBs, and their post-procedure pain scores were reduced.

Park's observational study added to the previous findings of Engelmann and colleagues in 2011, who conducted a randomised controlled trial (RCT) of complex laparoscopic surgeries performed in the conventional way or with "intermittent pneumoperitoneum" (i.e. taking breaks from operating).[93] They showed that taking breaks reduced intraoperative events and physiological stress levels, as shown by 22%

lower serum cortisol levels, and decreased alpha-amylase levels in the surgeons' saliva. Those surgeons taking breaks from operating also had a pre- to post-operative increase in error rate on a concentration test four times lower than in those surgeons randomised to conventional operating. Crucially, as in Park's study this RCT found that taking breaks didn't prolong the duration of the operations. Breaks pay for themselves. In combination with our anecdotal experiences of feeling better when we stop even briefly, these studies strongly favour taking breaks when possible.

Related to the benefits of taking breaks is the time they afford us to top up our glucose levels, a nutritional replenishment that has also been shown to fight decision fatigue. Researchers from Ben Gurion University of the Negev in Israel and Columbia Business School in New York found that judges making decisions on whether to accept or reject prisoners' applications for parole exhibited clear evidence of decision fatigue.[94] The percentage of parole applications accepted dropped from approximately 65% at the start of a session to almost zero right before a meal break was due, and then returned to baseline at the start of the next "decision session". Just like the NHS Scotland nurses staffing the helpline, the rising decision fatigue pushed the judges towards the default option, which in this case was to reject the parole application and keep the prisoner behind bars, guaranteeing public safety. This 2011 paper has become one of the most well-known demonstrations of decision fatigue. But was it only the break from deciding that helped the judges' decision-making return to baseline, or were the calories consumed at the mealtime also playing a role?

Experiments in the Baumeister lab found that sugar-containing lemonade, but not a control drink containing diet sweetener, had the capacity to restore participants' willpower after it had been depleted. Subsequently, a study in which 45 female dieters had their willpower reduced by watching a comedy film without laughing, before being shown images of appetising food, found that inducing mental fatigue caused increased reward centre activation in the brain's nucleus accumbens and decreased impulse control activity in the amygdala in response to the food images, as shown on functional brain imaging. However, these effects were completely reversible with the administration of glucose. The results offered a neurobiological explanation for the ability of sugar to reverse the impacts of mental fatigue, even though total brain energy consumption remained relatively constant. When willpower had been depleted, the brain had become more focused on short-term rewards (with increased nucleus accumbens activation), a change that could drive the decision-fatigue shortcuts we have discussed: rapid heuristics, decision avoidance or taking the easy default option. These all come with a potential cost to decision quality. Given the importance of stable blood glucose levels for combatting decision fatigue, we should try to eat low glycaemic index, healthy meals ideally before midnight on the night shift, giving our metabolism the best shot at supporting our decisions.

Although this chapter about safety at night seemed a natural home for a discussion of decision fatigue, decision fatigue can occur on any long shift, particularly out-of-hours, when we could accumulate mental and emotional strain from a high burden of decision-making. It is just that on night shifts, with an increased burden of higher-stakes decisions and the added factor of our tiredness at play, we are particularly vulnerable. Some will inevitably suggest that the most junior doctors do not, and more importantly should not, make the most important decisions, so do they really need to worry so much about decision fatigue? This argument is flawed, even without considering that today's junior doctors are tomorrow's senior ones. As addressed in Chapter 1, new doctors constantly have to decide if they can decide alone, or whether they need to bump a decision up the chain. When working at night with skeleton staffing, very few decisions are automatically escalated, so even at the bottom of the chain the risks are high.

Almost all doctors will recognise the experience of feeling dangerously fatigued, and you would be forgiven for feeling that this chapter has so far made for gloomy reading regarding the acutely unwell patients we look after at night, the higher rates of medical error and the adverse effects of fatigue on our clinical thinking. However, we have already seen how deliberately restricting our decision-making, taking sensible breaks and micro-breaks, and aiming for stable blood glucose levels can reduce levels of decision fatigue. And across a set of night shifts, there are further steps we can take to mitigate the risks. If we better understand the sleep science and physiology of the night shift cycle, we can handle the challenge, feel good in ourselves and give safer care to our patients.

The Night Shift Cycle

Strategies and techniques for coping with night shifts are common topics of conversation in hospital staff rooms and the doctors' mess. Many theories abound, but some are more accurate than others. One common misconception is that we "flip" our body clocks when we do a set of nights. "The first night shift is a bit rough," they'll say confidently, "but once I've synced into night mode I'll be totally fine." It would be nice if this was true, but unfortunately it is a myth. In *Why We Sleep*, Professor Matthew Walker explains that when he flies east from San Francisco to London, the sunlight signals to the brain's suprachiasmatic nucleus mean that he will eventually overcome the jet lag, but the process is slow.[95] Much too slow. "For every day you are in a different time zone," he writes, "your suprachiasmatic nucleus can only adjust by about one hour." For a doctor who is staying awake longer than their usual circadian rhythm is expecting as they come onto night shifts, our equivalent of rapidly flying east through multiple time zones, there is no hope of circadian re-synchronisation coming to our rescue. We will have finished our run of night shifts before the process is even halfway done.

The body clock flipping believers are right about one thing though – the first night shift usually does feel the roughest. This common observation actually has to do with 'sleep pressure', the second determinant of wakefulness, which together with the internal circadian rhythm governs whether or not we feel alert, fired up and ready to go. In sleep physiology, these two key factors are referred to as 'Process-C' (for circadian wake drive) and 'Process-S' (for sleep pressure), which is mediated by accumulating levels of adenosine in the brain. Over the course of a normal 24-hour period, Process-C and Process-S work in tandem to keep us awake when we should be awake, and to help us sleep when we should sleep (Figure 4.2). In the morning, Process-C is ramping up and cortisol levels are increasing, combining with the low levels of sleep pressure at this early stage of the day to mean that we are appropriately wakeful. When the distance between Process-S and Process-C is small, there is a strong urge to stay awake. Then, as the day wears on and Process-C turns the corner, decreasing the circadian wake drive, and sleep pressure continues to build as our hours awake accumulate, the distance between the two grows until eventually we fall asleep. Sleep washes out the accumulated adenosine, reducing Process-S back down until, sometime after the circadian tide turns at its nadir around 4 am, the distance between Process-S and Process-C is small enough that we wake up and begin the cycle once more.

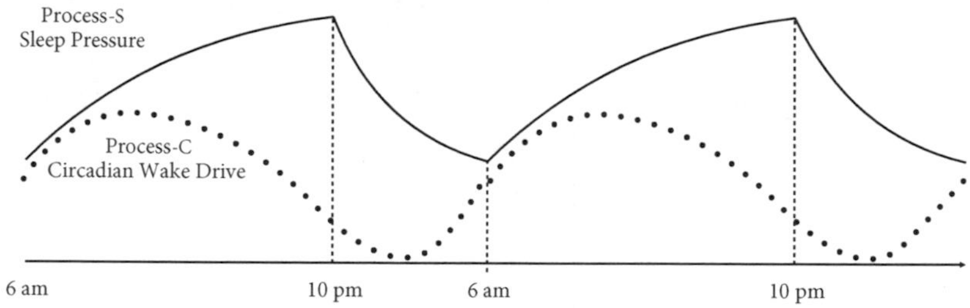

Figure 4.2 The two-process model of sleep. Process-C (circadian wake drive) and Process-S (sleep pressure in the biochemical form of brain adenosine levels) are the two opposing forces regulating whether we feel awake or sleepy. (After Borbély, 1982.)

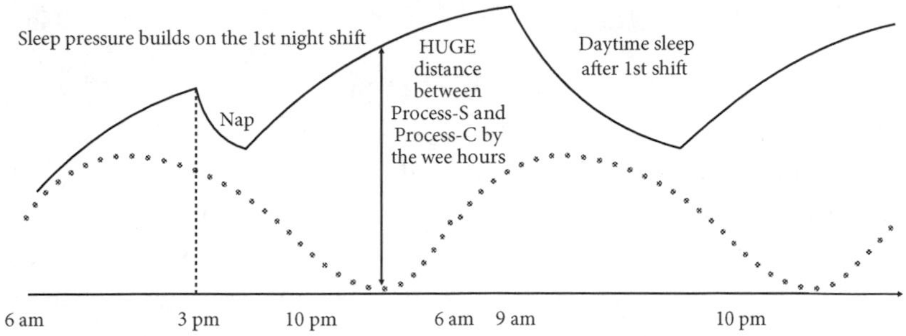

Figure 4.3 The night shift cycle. Our feeling of fatigue when working at night, determined by the gap between Process-C and Process-S, reaches its maximum point in the wee hours of the morning. Although the gap narrows with the morning rise in Process-C, giving the 'second wind', the sleep pressure curve continues to build until eventually it is overwhelming.

Now consider what happens as we head into the night shift cycle (Figure 4.3). You can probably see where this is heading. As we begin the first night shift, Process-S will be on the way up, even if we have managed a successful nap that afternoon. Process-C, meanwhile, is on the way down towards its lowest point. For a 9 pm to 9 am night shift, this means that the distance between Process-S and Process-C will constantly be increasing for the first part of the shift, progressively lowering our wakefulness. It is this high burden of accumulating sleep pressure, rather than circadian de-synchronisation, which makes the first night shift feel the worst. The interplay between Process-C and Process-S also explains two night shift phenomena that most doctors will recognise anecdotally: 'the witching hour' or 'hitting the wall' around 4 am, and the 'second wind' as the sun starts to rise and the light cues (zeitgebers) from outside combine with the re-booting circadian wake drive to temporarily let us feel and function better, despite having been awake and working for longer overall.

Navigating the Nights

This map of the night shift cycle prompts a few suggestions about how we can optimise performance and reduce the chances of making mistakes. Firstly, the major contribution of Process-S on the first night shift underlines the importance of not doing anything particularly mentally or physically taxing on the day of the shift, and of trying to get some sleep in the afternoon. On one occasion when I didn't get any afternoon sleep before nights, the difference I noticed on the shift was frightening. I had spent the morning doing online revision questions due to an upcoming exam, hadn't done very well with them and then couldn't sleep that afternoon. This meant that I was starting the night shift having already been awake for more than 12 hours. By 4 am, 'hitting the wall' was an understatement. I was catastrophically tired, with even the most basic decisions taking three, four, five times as much mental effort as usual. Fortunately, I realised what was happening, double-checked everything and limited myself to only the absolutely necessary decisions until the sun was rising and the circadian boost could get me through until handover.

Even if we are well-rested before a night shift, maintaining awareness that we will hit our physiological nadir around 4 am warns us to be extra-careful with anything we are doing at this stage of the night. Roy Baumeister puts it like this – "The best decision makers are the ones who know when not to trust themselves." The now-established understanding of sleep physiology means that we have a scientific basis for what more senior doctors have appreciated from experience and gut instinct over the years. "I'm convinced there's a witching hour where you almost have to deal with that demon inside you that says things will be fine, just go back to bed," stated Professor Peter Brindley on the *Mastering Intensive Care* podcast.[96] "That normalcy bias that can exist in the daytime is even more so at night-time," he added. This idea of normalcy bias worsening at night is closely related to the ability of decision fatigue to drive us towards the default option. If our default belief is always that the patient will be fine, or that we can safely 'continue current management', we risk missing the signs of a deteriorating patient and the opportunity to intervene.

One other consideration is the role of something that doctors seem to like talking about almost as much as they like drinking – coffee. Caffeine, described by Matthew Walker as "the most widely used (and abused) psychoactive stimulant in the world"[97], competes with adenosine for binding sites at its receptors in the brain, giving it the ability to stave off sleep pressure and boost alertness. It is only a temporary roadblock for Process-S though, rather than a reversal agent. With time, the caffeine is metabolised by liver cytochrome P450 enzymes, freeing up brain receptor space for the sleep-inducing adenosine that has continued to accumulate. Therefore, if we drink coffee near the start of a night shift, we should be aware of the potential for a 'caffeine crash' when the effects wear off. It is also important to avoid a morning coffee on the day of the first night shift, to maximise the chances of a successful pre-nights nap in the afternoon. Similarly, caffeine should be avoided in the last few hours of the night shift since we need as much daytime sleep as possible. This comes with the caveat, however, that a shot of caffeine may be required if we need to drive home safely, something we will return to at the end of the chapter. Overall, the use of coffee can help get us through the night shift cycle, but we should almost treat it as a prescription drug; careless consumption outside of the advisable timings or quantities has the potential to make things worse.

A non-exhaustive set of suggestions to help navigate the nights is shown in Box 4.1, inspired by a BMJ review article by McKenna and Wilkes.[98]

BOX 4.1 A RANGE OF SIMPLE, SENSIBLE STEPS AT THE VARIOUS STAGES OF THE NIGHT SHIFT CYCLE CAN HELP US MINIMISE THE RISKS

BEFORE THE FIRST NIGHT

Goal: Minimise sleep debt

- Don't set an alarm for that morning
- No caffeine that morning
- Nap in the afternoon, ideally in multiples of 90 minutes (one sleep cycle)

DURING THE NIGHTS

Goal: Patient safety

- Plan breaks with your team
- Create self-checks for safety-critical tasks, e.g. prescribing potassium, insulin or anticoagulants
- Beware the witching hour

BETWEEN THE NIGHTS

Goal: Minimise sleep debt

- Apply basic sleep hygiene – no alcohol, limit screen time
- Invest in blackout blinds or blackout curtains, or try an eye-mask
- If you wake up and can't sleep, get up for a short while but then try to sleep again

POST-NIGHTS

Goal: Return to normality*

- Sleep early, for either 3 or 4.5 hours
- Get up. This can be unpleasant. Hang on in there.
- Go outside and walk around
- Go to bed at a normal person's bedtime

* If you are on an ED rota, consider "normality" a relative term.

The Second Wind

We have seen in the night shift cycle how our physiology conspires against us around 4 am, often causing an overwhelming feeling of tiredness when we have been going for 8 hours and the end doesn't seem to be anywhere in sight. Fortunately, the turning of the circadian tide and the ramping up of Process-C comes to our rescue. Very often it feels like this is just in time. I have absolutely no scientific basis for this, but there always seems to be a surprising volume of bleeps around 6 am. Maybe it's because that's when the previously well patients' 4-hourly observations are done, and it turns out things are not as stable as before. I can find myself in full flow around 6.30 or 7 am, assessing patients with a clarity of thought that would have been impossible a couple of hours earlier. It is the light cues coming through the hospital windows and the narrowing of the distance between Process-C and Process-S that gives us this capacity.

Early one morning on the AMU, just a couple of hours away from finishing an exhausting run of four nights, the nurses asked me to urgently clerk Deepali, a 19-year-old woman who was feeling short of breath. Her chart stated that she was requiring a couple of litres of oxygen to maintain her saturations, and her heart rate and respiratory rate were high. I rapidly scanned the available information. Deepali had no past medical history at all – she was a normally fit and well economics student at university. The ED team had started her on antibiotics for a possible chest infection and had also raised the possibility of asthma. However, the inflammatory markers in her blood were totally normal, and she had no fevers. Deepali told me she had a slight nagging pain beneath her right breast, but she did not have a cough, her breathing was not worse at night, she did not have any history of eczema or allergies, and nothing like this had ever happened before. She had not travelled anywhere, had no pets and took no regular medications.

As I began to examine her, I realised that her vital signs could not be the same as those I had seen on her paper chart. Her radial pulse felt quick, very quick, surely more than the 105 beats per minute previously recorded. She was speaking in short sentences, with her respiratory rate visibly high. Even more concerning was her respiratory pattern, the left side of her chest rising and falling smoothly, but totally out-of-kilter with the right side of the chest, which didn't seem to be moving much at all. I listened, quickly. There was no wheeze to suggest asthma and no crackles to suggest fluid or infection, only an unnerving quietness on the right-hand side. Despite the accumulated fatigue of the past four nights, my brain was moving quickly now, eliminating the possible diagnoses Deepali had arrived with from the ED. There was no way this was acute asthma or a chest infection. I percussed the right side of Deepali's chest. It was hyper-resonant.

I ducked out of the cubicle and fetched an observations machine, popping the saturations probe on Deepali's finger and fitting the blood pressure cuff. My suspicions were confirmed, with her heart racing at 145 beats per minute and her respiratory rate at 36. Worse still, the blue number from the sats probe stared back at me – 85%. Young people have a remarkable ability to compensate for profound disturbances for hours on end as their strong physiological reserve rises to the challenge, but the eventual decompensation can be dramatic. Deepali was heading in the wrong direction.

"Gina, can I have some help in here please?" I called through the thin blue curtains. "Can we have the non-rebreathe mask?" Gina was one of the best nurses in the AMU and had the mask for Deepali within seconds, but it was no good. Her oxygen levels still wouldn't go higher than 91%. I picked up the nurses' station phone, hit 2222 and called the crash team. As the buzzer blared and the resuscitation trolley was wheeled into the bedspace, Deepali looked confused – were things really that bad? I thought that they very soon might be. Less than an hour before she had only needed 2 litres of oxygen, and now her saturations were just 91% despite the 15 litres of oxygen we were giving her. She was not ventilating her right lung at all and was in respiratory failure.

Steve, the night registrar, arrived, shortly followed by Rachel the ICU registrar, and I explained what was going on. The portable chest

X-ray team came next, and we saw the image on the monitor of their machine. Whilst the left lung field looked normal, the right side of the chest was mostly filled with an empty black space. Deepali had an enormous pneumothorax. Her vital signs remained precarious, and Rachel made the decision to take Deepali upstairs to the thoracic HDU for an emergency chest drain.

Now that Deepali was in safe hands, I retreated back to the AMU office. Not for the first time, the second wind at the end of the night had come to my rescue, and to Deepali's. With a healthy shot of adrenaline from seeing her deranged observations and the diagnostic tool of time passing, I had been able to avoid the diagnosis momentum bias as it became apparent that things were not what they had first seemed. The day team arrived. "How was the night?" the consultant asked. "It all got a bit busy at the end there," I replied. With the arrival of the daytime doctors, we could finally hand over to fresher minds and know that our turn was done. It had been a really challenging run of nights. But even at this stage of a shift, as the dust starts to settle on the highs and lows of the night, we still have one more safety-critical task to do. We need to get home.

Safely Home

Shortly before 9 am on the 3rd of August 2015, Dr Ronak Patel was driving home after his shift, the third in a set of nights on-call as a trainee anaesthetist at the Norfolk and Norwich University Hospital. He was very tired, but understandably was anxious to get home to his wife, Helen. Aware that he needed to stay awake, Ronak called Helen on the hands-free set, and they sang songs to try and keep him awake on the drive. Then the line cut out. Helen re-dialled several times, but there was no reply. Unable to stave off the grip of his fatigue, Ronak had fallen asleep and his car had drifted out of lane, into the path of an oncoming lorry. His neck was broken, and he was declared dead at the scene.[99]

I first heard the harrowing story of Dr Patel's death during a teaching session about wellbeing, fatigue and working at night. My colleagues and I had been shocked into silence as we heard what had happened. However, when presented with tragedies of this kind there is a tendency to assume that because they are rare, they will not happen to us. We feel stunned and sad upon hearing the story, but the perception that fatal accidents are rare means that we may not attribute them sufficient importance to actually change our behaviour. Instead, we soon become re-occupied with immediate concerns on the wards, with exams or deadlines, with our lives outside the hospital, or simply with wondering what's for lunch. Knowledge of rare events, however shocking, can drift from our attention. It was only when I read more about Ronak in the national newspaper reports from the time, learning that he had grown up just ten miles from my family home and, like me, had travelled to New Zealand to gain experience and gone on to choose a career in anaesthetics, that the reality of what had happened to him really hit home. Ronak's story could have been any of ours.

So far, I have avoided giving too many direct pieces of advice in this book. It is not intended to be specific instructions – getting things right as a new doctor is often more complicated than "if x then do y". However, the general policy of avoiding prescriptive advice will now be (temporarily) suspended. When it's time to get home from night shifts, you really should not drive if you can possibly avoid it. In *Why We Sleep*, Matthew Walker is particularly strong on this issue, pointing out experiments showing that sleep deprivation from being awake for 19 hours produces a level of cognitive impairment equalling that seen in subjects who were legally drunk. Research has also found that the risk of a car crash increases exponentially for every hour of sleep lost.[100] As Walker argues, "To carry the burden of another's death on your shoulders is a terrible thing" and driving when dangerously tired is "just not worth the (life) cost"[101].

I have friends and colleagues who have fallen asleep at the wheel on the way home, thankfully damaging no more than their own car.

I know many more who admit to momentarily drifting into a 'micro-sleep' whilst driving, jolting awake and realising what they have done. It is a terrifying prospect. The impression of serious risk from these anecdotes is born out in large surveys, with the Royal College of Anaesthetists finding in 2017 that 57% of the 2231 UK trainee anaesthetists who responded had had an accident or near-miss on the journey home after a night shift.[102] Considering that these data are from doctors in just one speciality, there must be thousands risking their own and others' lives in fatigue-induced incidents on the roads.

Notably, a further survey published in *Anaesthesia* in 2019, focused this time on consultants, suggested that the risks of commuting whilst fatigued are at their highest in the first stage of our careers, during the trainee years.[103] Of the 3847 consultant anaesthetists and paediatric intensivists in the UK and Republic of Ireland who responded (a response rate of 46%), 45% admitted to having had an accident or near miss commuting whilst fatigued. Importantly, 72% of these incidents occurred back when the individual was a trainee, and another 15% reported an accident or near miss both as a trainee and as a consultant. These data can't be explained away by only a relatively young selection of consultants responding to the survey either; 78% of respondents had been working as a consultant for at least six years. Whilst the findings are not surprising given that it is trainee doctors who provide the majority of night cover and regular rotation between hospitals means that we tend to have longer commutes, they serve as a reminder for us all. It is in the years when we are most junior that we are most vulnerable to the potentially deadly effects of fatigue.

For those living and working in major cities, it may be relatively simple to take public transport home at the end of the night, making it easy to do the right thing for both our own safety and the safety of others. Yet in regions where commuting distances are longer, with fewer transport links, we may feel as though we have no option but to drive home – we can't sleep in the hospital car park. In fact, in the 2016 junior doctors' contract there is an obligation on the part of the employer to provide employees who feel too tired to safely travel home after a night shift or a long, late shift with either an appropriate rest facility in which to sleep or, failing that, to arrange alternative travel home. Although this obligation exists in writing, it is not often publicised. To keep doctors and their patients safe, hospitals need to develop straightforward and simple systems to access rest spaces or transport home.

In their article about optimising sleep for night shifts, McKenna and Wilkes comment, “responsibility for maintaining worker health and performance is shared between organisations and workers”. In this chapter we have explored in detail what the individual worker can and should be doing to maximise their performance and so enhance patient safety at night, but not all hospitals are keeping their half of the bargain. Very often there is no provision of hot food overnight and there is nowhere to take structured rest breaks. It is also uncommon to find a transparent and easily accessible system in place for trainees to access their contractual entitlement to rest facilities or transport home when they are too exhausted to drive safely. Perhaps McKenna and Wilkes’ statement might be revised to say that responsibility *should* be shared. At present in the UK, the responsibility for managing the risks of fatigue to both patients and to doctors themselves is born squarely by the doctors in the hospital at night.

In Chapter 5, we take a change of pace and consider some of the issues for new doctors caring for patients at the end of their lives. Up until now we have discussed patient safety almost entirely from the perspective of avoiding morbidity and mortality – trying to stop people from getting any sicker or from dying. Yet a significant part of our work is looking after patients who we cannot make better, those who *are* dying. What does it mean to keep somebody safe from harm in his or her final weeks, days or hours of life? As new doctors, our greatest involvement in this area is likely to occur out-of-hours, or in the early hours, when there are fewer senior staff around to help. How should we prepare to become a patient’s final doctor?

"When a disease insinuates itself so potently into the imagination of an era, it is often because it impinges on an anxiety latent within that imagination. . . . Society, like the ultimate psychosomatic patient, matches its medical afflictions to its psychological crises; when a disease touches such a visceral chord, it is often because that chord is already resonating."

Siddhartha Mukherjee, *The Emperor of All Maladies*

INTERLUDE

GOING VIRAL

After I finished my ICU rotation on the University Spaceship, I switched jobs and joined the Microbiology Department. The extensive and detailed knowledge of pathogenic bacteria that microbiology doctors require in order to give advice to other teams meant that this was a placement designed almost entirely for educational purposes; my role was to be helpful to the team and learn everything I could along the way. I had been qualified for 16 months now and life was good. The registrars and consultants teaching me were approachable and kind, we were helping look after some interesting patients and, amazingly, my job for the next four months was scheduled as Monday to Friday, 9 am to 5 pm. I was enjoying the novelty. I worked in an office with the registrars, where teams would phone through their microbiological queries, which we would sift through and investigate on the online patient information system, often before going to see the patient on the ward. We were getting into the work one morning when Frieda came in. "Have a read of this, Luke," she said brightly. "It's about a novel coronavirus that's been detected in Wuhan Province in China." Dr Frieda Christiansen was one of the consultant virologists who worked in the same office as we did. "Thanks a lot," I said, wanting to be polite. "I'll take a look at it."

In fact, I didn't think novel coronaviruses sounded especially exciting. I was much more interested in bacteria and the severe sepsis and critical illness they could trigger. As part of the microbiology rotation, I had recently spent a couple of days in the bacteriology laboratory with Steven, one of the expert biomedical scientists who had more than 20 years' experience identifying pathogenic bacteria from their appearances down the microscope. He was very patient with my clumsy attempts at performing a Gram stain, but we succeeded eventually and together examined slides of *Neisseria meningitidis*, prepared from the blood cultures of a critically unwell patient I had helped look after when covering a shift on the ICU the day before. It was a moment of bench-to-bedside clinical correlation that is exceedingly rare in medical training nowadays. My interest was piqued, and for the next few weeks I carried on trying to learn about infection and also worked on audits concerning antibiotic prescribing for major surgery and central line infections in the ICU. The paper about the novel coronavirus sat under a pile of others on my desk, unread and forgotten.

Less than 12 weeks later, on 6 April 2020, I stood in blue scrubs outside the ICU, beneath a temporary sign declaring 'Donning Station'. I gelled my hands and tied on a theatre cap. Now I needed a surgical gown. Were there any that weren't either large or extra-large? No. "Oh well, at least we've got something," I thought, remembering pictures on the news of staff elsewhere fashioning gowns out of bin bags. I pulled it on and a theatre nurse helped me tie the ties up at the back. She was helping here because every single elective operation had been cancelled. Next, a respirator mask. I bent the top tightly over the bridge of my nose to ensure a good seal, and blew out twice, hard, to check air was not leaking around the sides. For eye protection, I picked up a plastic face shield and pulled the elastic round the back of my head. This would be better than the goggles, I reasoned, since it would stop me absent-mindedly touching my face. Lastly, I put on two pairs of gloves. Debbie, one of the Critical Care research nurses I knew appeared besides me as she completed the donning procedure. She had been rushed back to clinical practice having been working in research for the past four years. We stretched and flexed in the alien outfits we now found ourselves in, walking uneasily towards the double doors in our oversized gowns.

> "I'm scared, Luke," Debbie confided.
>
> "Yes, me too," I replied. "But we do have good teams here. We'll manage somehow."
>
> The doors opened, we passed beneath a second sign and entered the Covid-ICU.

The rapidly unfolding events of early 2020 that led from the novel coronavirus being an unread academic paper on my desk to my redeployment to ICU amidst an almost apocalyptic scenario as coronavirus swept across the UK have already been well-documented and described. Both Rachel Clarke in *Breathtaking: Inside the NHS in a Time of Pandemic*[104] and Dominic Pimenta in *Duty of Care: One NHS Doctor's Story of Courage and Compassion on the COVID-19 Frontline*[105] precisely capture the growing anxiety and disbelief amongst the medical profession as the UK government needlessly delayed the inevitable lockdown and failed to take sufficient measures to protect both those who would land in the ICU on a ventilator and the vulnerable people in hospices, care homes and the wider community. *Failures of State: The Inside Story of Britain's Battle with Coronavirus* chronicles the government's serial negligence with devastating clarity.[106] Just over 100 years after the Spanish flu of 1918, the consequence of a pandemic played out in the digital age is that the data and stories which map its causes, course and consequences have been shared faster and more widely, for all to see.

Sometimes the stories that are told from significant events in our lives are notable in their uniqueness, memorable by their singularity. They stand out because they are so dramatically different and abnormal. And for us as individuals, our experiences inside the Covid-ICU are precisely that. They fit this bill. When I walked through those double doors, it was surreal, like entering into a disaster movie. Caring for row upon row of critically unwell patients, all struck down by the same disease and dehumanised by what we had done trying to save them from it, was like nothing we could have imagined. Yet the tragedy was that what I experienced was *not* remotely unique. In every city across the country the same storylines were playing out again and again: patients plunging into respiratory failure terrified and alone, facing certain death or a 50/50 chance of survival on the ventilator, overcrowded ICUs stretched to double or beyond double their normal capacity, nurses and doctors pushed to breaking point, the hardest of telephone calls to patients' families often muffled through layers of PPE, and the steeliness and resolve that kept all our teams working day after night after day after night through it all. Our stories of Covid-19 are frightening by their ubiquity.

Rather than narrating the chronology of my own and others' experiences of Covid-19 and attempting to draw lessons from it, which could imply a clearly defined end to the pandemic, we need to consider the remaining issues of this book in the new context in which we find ourselves. Equally, in our discussion of how new doctors can get things right, we do not need a chapter about the safety of 'The Covid-19 patient', since all the principles we have encountered so far apply as much, and probably more, in coronavirus wards and within healthcare systems stretched past their limits by a pandemic. And the topics that comprise the second half of this book, including care of the dying patient, thinking about our own wellbeing in order to properly look after others, and wayfinding through the complex and often uncertain early stages of our lives and careers cannot in any meaningful sense be discussed in the setting of a pre-Covid world.

The emergence of SARS-CoV-2 has changed everything, and at the time of writing the expert consensus suggests that it is here to stay. Even if we are successful in updating the current vaccines as new variants arise, reaching an uncomfortable but manageable equilibrium in this virus versus vaccine arms race and limiting further Covid-19 mortality to levels that society deems acceptable, there is no way of truly returning to the world that we knew in late 2019. Whether you are reading this as a student in college or university, a young doctor starting out, a senior doctor who supervises us or as an interested citizen, we have all by necessity changed too much and learned too much across the course of the pandemic to continue our discussion any further in its absence. Despite its 200-nanometre diameter, SARS-CoV-2 would have been the largest of all elephants in the room. The following pages are therefore set squarely in the pandemic world.

"So let us not talk falsely now,
The hour is getting late."

Bob Dylan, *All Along the Watchtower*

5

THEIR FINAL DOCTOR

CARING FOR PATIENTS AT THE END

Safe Passage on Your Travels

So far in *The Bleep Test*, we have looked into a range of areas relating to keeping patients safe, focusing on how we can avoid making errors and help things go right. We have mainly considered patient safety through the lens of recognising, managing and escalating the deteriorating hospital inpatient – bluntly, trying to ensure that sick patients do not die. Because doctoring is about saving lives, isn't it? But what about the times when the patient is not getting better despite our treatments, when they have reached the ceiling of their care and they *are* dying? The definition of patient safety we came across in Chapter 1 refers to the avoidance of preventable harm, and there is plenty of potential for harm in the care of the dying and the dead, and the heartbroken and the bereaved. We need to recognise the point when our interventions are not working and are only compromising dignity and comfort, communicate empathetically with patients and their loved ones, treat distressing symptoms and support families at the end. Here, too, there is deep water for us to swim in.

When I was in medical school, I had (perhaps naively) thought that the work of recognising irreversible deterioration in a dying patient, trying to ensure they did not suffer, breaking the bad news to their families and continuing to communicate with them throughout the process would be skills for later, and not for the first year of clinical practice. However, I soon found that in the evenings or at night, especially in surgical rotations when the registrar could be needed in theatre for hours, there was only me. In caring for the dying patient, as in so much of medical training, the paradox is that it is usually when we are most stretched and alone that we are required to practise right at the upper end of our ability.

There will be those who will protest at this point that these scenarios should never happen, that new doctors should never have to manage a patient at the end of their life or be the only doctor present to tell relatives that the person they love most in all the world is dying or has died. However, rigidly following a 'fully supported and supervised at all times' mantra for new doctors' training is both ignoring the real world of staffing and service pressures and missing the more fundamental point that the moment the first year is up and we become SHOs, we will be expected to deal with common end-of-life issues relatively independently. And as Covid-19 swept across the world in early 2020, hospitals were confronted with overwhelming numbers of dying patients needing end-of-life care. There were deaths occurring on a scale that would previously have been unimaginable. So how can we best look after patients when we are at once a new doctor and their final doctor?

Advocating

One autumnal Tuesday morning, a newly qualified doctor called Sachin was doing the ward round in the stroke unit with his consultant, Dr Jones, and the rest of the team. Sachin was finding it a tricky placement, with complex patients who needed weeks of rehabilitation to try and recover some of the function they had lost. Medical school had focused mainly on acute stroke management, but it was only now – doing the job for real – that he was beginning to appreciate the devastating effects of a stroke and the efforts of the patients trying to recover. Not all of them did. Sachin was learning in this, his first job, to come to terms with some of his patients dying.

The ward round arrived at Bay 3 and reached Bob, a 79-year-old retired postman who had suffered a major stroke affecting the whole right side of his body, his ability to speak and, dangerously, his ability to swallow. The therapists on the ward did not think Bob would be able to swallow food safely, so the conversation amongst the staff gathered around the computer at the foot of Bob's bed turned quickly to feeding options, specifically when would be the first available opportunity to get a tube inserted into Bob's stomach. Bob was still finding speaking very slow going, so when this plan was hastily communicated to him, Sachin couldn't shake the feeling that Bob hadn't really been given the chance to have his say.

Sachin lightly touched the shoulder of Jenny, the other newly qualified doctor on the team, and gestured discretely back towards the slightly distressed-looking Bob. "Give me 15 minutes and I'll catch you up," he said. Jenny nodded. It was reassuring how the two of them always seemed to be on the same wavelength. Once the ward round was done and everyone sat down in the office for the daily meeting, Sachin worked up the courage to pass on what he'd learned in those 15 minutes.

"Bob understands that the food might go down the wrong way and end up in his lungs, and that it could cause him to get pneumonia and even die," Sachin told Dr Jones. "But it's what he wants to do. He and his wife have cooked and eaten together for the last 58 years. He can't bear the thought of artificial feeding. Going home and at least *trying* to eat is what's important to him."

Dr Jones replied:

> Oh, thanks for taking the time to sit with Bob and find that out, Sachin. I hadn't realised he had thought about the feeding issue and thought so much about the risks. I'll go back and talk to him properly and, if he's sure, we can do a feeding at risk form and get him home. We can hold off on booking the PEG.

Bob was sure, it turned out, and Sachin did the discharge paperwork later that afternoon. Hospital transport arrived just before 5 pm and got Bob home safely, with some (softened) roast dinner waiting for him and not an item of feeding equipment in sight.

Stories like this remind us that new doctors are not simply partially trained, non-specialist 'doctor-light' versions of their registrars and consultants. Being the most junior doctor in a team is a unique role we will occupy only once in our careers, one which, despite the numerous challenges, brings with it a different perspective and position from which to advocate for patients. "The first-year doctor is probably the closest to the patient of anyone on the team," argued Sachin, now a few years into his surgical training. "They are on the wards the most and can see what is happening on a daily basis. They can bring information to their seniors after conversations with patients that can help convey a patient's wishes."

When it comes to caring for patients who are gravely sick and may not survive, it can sometimes be a direct product of our medical inexperience that we can excel and help everyone to get things right. As new doctors, we will not have the best prescribing, diagnostic or surgical skills on any team, but we are well placed to rank 1st for kindness, approachability, and ability to listen. "End-of-life care is one of the only times I feel like I'm doing a good job," one new doctor told a group gathered in the office. James, a friend from university, expanded on these sentiments, telling me, "Palliative care is probably one of the more rewarding parts of medicine. It feels very different from the rest of the job. It's entirely focused on just making people feel better." We should feel motivated and encouraged that palliative care is an area where new doctors can make an enormous difference to the care patients receive and the experience of their families.

Although there are more complex cases that require discussion with specialist palliative care teams, there are also plenty of cases that are (technically at least) relatively straightforward, where patients' symptoms can be managed with a routine set of prescriptions. In hospital end-of-life care, it can often be the non-technical aspects that are the most challenging part. If we do not handle these issues well there is the potential to cause harm, but we also have a huge opportunity to get things right. In situations that are full of sadness and tragedy and grief, it is our privilege to be in a position to help things be handled as well as they could be in those circumstances. Breaking bad news to a patient or their loved ones is one of the most important tasks in this work.

Breaking Bad News

What does it mean to break bad news? 'Bad news' has been defined as "any information which adversely and seriously affects an individual's view of his or her future"[107]. But do we really need a definition for what counts as bad news? At first glance what counts as 'bad news' seems obvious, but this definition does bring up a couple of important points. Firstly, it reminds us that revealing a grave diagnosis signals not only the beginning of a period dealing with the immediate medical consequences of the news (e.g. starting chemotherapy), but also the loss of a previously anticipated future. In the space of seconds, the myriad possible lives the patient or their loved ones had viewed as open doors are slammed shut. The bad news rips away those futures and ensures they will never happen. Often while the grim medical reality is still playing out, they are already grieving for those moments that are lost.

Secondly, we can infer that *how* bad the news is depends on *how much* it changes that person's view of their future. What is the gap between their expectations (based on prior knowledge and understanding) and the reality we are about to reveal? If, for example, we are telling a patient who already knows they have metastatic colon cancer that their most recent CT scan shows an increase in the number of liver metastases, that bad news does not radically alter their view of their future in the same way as their initial diagnosis would have done. Although it is never easy, in this scenario the breaking bad news conversation only has to bridge the distance between the viewpoints of "I have metastatic colon cancer which has spread to my liver and is going to kill me" and "I have metastatic colon cancer which has spread to my liver and is going to kill me, and is getting worse despite the palliative chemotherapy I've been taking." This is still challenging news to deliver, but is more straightforward than the opposite situation where there is a gulf between a patient's expectations and the reality.

One evening on the General Medicine ward, the nurses asked me to talk to Tess, a 56-year-old woman, about the results of her CT head scan. She had presented with left arm weakness and pins and needles in her left hand, so the day team had requested the CT scan, worried that she had suffered a stroke. Tragically, the scan showed a large tumour that was most likely to be a Glioblastoma, a type of brain cancer that is usually aggressive and very, very bad news. "Shit," I thought. She was younger than my Mum and I was about to deliver what was probably a death sentence. I asked Sister Trudy to come with me to talk to Tess.

"Is there a consultation room on the ward we could use?" I asked her.

"I'm sorry, Luke, it has to be deep cleaned because one of the patients in there earlier turned out to be Covid positive," Trudy replied.

Sound proof blue curtains would have to do. We often seem to trade down and settle for the illusion of privacy.

"Does Tess have any family close by who could come in to be with her?"

"She lives alone, she has her sister, but I asked her earlier and she's three hours away . . . and even if she could get here, I'm not sure I could swing it with Matron . . . the Covid visiting rules say that families can only come in when a patient is end of life."

"Ok, let's go and talk to her."

Trudy and I walked into Bay 2, commandeered some plastic chairs from the other bed spaces and pulled the blue curtains around Tess's bed before sitting down.

"Hello. My name's Luke Austen, I'm one of the doctors looking after the ward this evening. Sister Trudy you've met already, I think."

"Ah yes, hello again, Trudy," Tess replied brightly. "Thanks for getting the evening doctor along. Is this about my CT scan results? The daytime doctor already told me that there was no stroke before he left, so can I be discharged home?"

Inside, my heart dropped like a stone. Trudy and I stole a horrified glance at one another. Tess had, in one short sentence, shown us her current understanding of her situation, and it couldn't be further from the truth. Worse still, the botched delivery of test results sharing the lack of any stroke but missing out the somewhat important fact of the large brain cancer had just made our task of breaking the bad news ten times harder. I tried to suppress my anger and incredulity at the daytime doctor. They were of no use now. *She thinks she's going home tonight. She thinks the scan is all clear.* I searched desperately for a way to bring Tess even slightly closer to the reality before breaking the news.

"I've just taken over from the day team this evening, Tess, and although I've read your notes, tell me from your perspective what was it that caused you to come into hospital? Talk me through what's happened so far."

"Well, doc, it's been going on a few weeks actually . . . the weakness I mean. Usually I'm fit as a fiddle, but I've been struggling to get my left arm to do what I tell it to. It had kind of crept up on me, if you know what I mean, but these last few days it really got bad. I was dropping things and started getting pins and needles in my left hand too."

"That sounds like things were definitely changing with your arm," I offered. "I'm sure you did the right thing coming in to get it investigated. Did you have any other symptoms?"

"Not really . . . except the headaches. I'm not a headache kind of person doc, but for the last week or so, it's definitely been there, especially first thing in the mornings. All a bit strange."

"Ok, so you were worried . . . and the team downstairs decided to do a CT head scan . . . did they tell you what they were looking for?"

"Ah yes, they said they thought I might have had a stroke, and that if it was a big stroke it would show up on the CT scan, but if it was only a small stroke, I might need an MRI."

"That's right, sometimes people do need MRI scans too," I said. "So, they'd mentioned stroke was one possibility . . . was there anything else you'd thought about what with this weakness and the headaches you'd been having?"

"I'd heard about strokes quite a bit on TV and did think I was a bit too young and fit to be having one," Tess replied. "I know it sounds crazy, doc, but I worried if it could be a tumour or something. But your colleague, the other guy, he told me already, there's no stroke on the CT scan, right?"

I paused.

"Tess . . ." I slowed down now, looking straight at her. "That's right, there's no sign of a stroke . . . but there is bad news on the CT scan report." I wait. Wait a second longer.

"Oh . . ." Tess sighed. "It's cancer, isn't it?"

"Yes – it does look that way. I'm so sorry to be bringing you this news." Now shut up, I tell myself. Be silent. Just be there, be here, for a few moments.

"How bad is it?" Tess asked.

"I'm no cancer doctor, but the consultant radiologist – the one who reported the CT scan – thinks that the images suggest quite an aggressive kind of brain cancer, Tess."

"So, it's bad bad."

"Yes, it's bad. I'm so sorry."

We sit in the stillness, and there is no noise coming from the other beds in the bay, or from the rest of the ward. Or maybe I have tuned it all out. A couple of silent tears roll down Tess's cheeks, as we sit with her in her shock. I see that Trudy brought along a box of tissues, but am glad that she has only placed them, without Tess ever noticing, within her reach. To offer them up to her or place one in her hand would only signal "Please, stop it! *We* are uncomfortable and would rather you stop crying." Instead, they are there when she is ready. Time is going in slow motion, and I guiltily think of all the other jobs on the ward I need to get back to. Wait, I tell myself. Just sit.

"So, what now?"

"I'm going to refer your case to the specialist Neuro team," I say. "In the meantime, we'll give you steroids to reduce the swelling around the tumour, and another tablet to protect your stomach lining from the steroids. We'll start with paracetamol for the headaches and can give you something more if you need it. I'll book you an urgent MRI for tomorrow so we can get a bit more information about what we're dealing with."

"Sounds like I won't be going home tonight then," Tess half chuckles. Many a true word said in jest.

"No, we do need to look after you here for now. . . . I'm sure this is a huge amount to take in, but Sister Trudy and I will be around if you want to talk. Is there anything else you want to ask me at the moment?"

"No . . . I'd better call my sister. Thank you for taking the time to tell me, doc."

"Not at all. Ok, I'll leave you for now. I'll do your referrals and MRI request before I finish tonight. See you later." I lift myself from the plastic chair and slip out of the blue curtains, leaving her behind in her radically altered world.

Telling Tess that her CT scan showed a brain cancer was an extremely challenging conversation, in part because of the gap we had to bridge between her false hope that had been created and the bad news we needed to tell her. Some might suggest that it shouldn't have been a junior doctor telling her this news. But it couldn't wait until morning – she needed the steroids to reduce the swelling as soon as possible, and she had a right to know why she was being handed those tablets rather than a discharge letter. I knew that the registrar was tied up with a couple of critically unwell patients on other wards, and I realised I *did* have the ability to break this news. In trying to deliver such a devastating diagnosis in the best way possible, I needed to draw on all the communication skills I had been trained in. However, it hasn't always been the case that doctors have been trained to think carefully about how they deliver bad news. In fact, they were previously encouraged to avoid telling patients bad news altogether.

"There was a lot of deception that went on around how sick people really were," said Dr Walter Baile on an episode of the *99 Percent Invisible* podcast discussing the history of breaking bad news.[108] "You couldn't talk about the patient dying, so you can imagine nobody really was able to say goodbye." This viewpoint was the mainstream. The podcast's host, Roman Mars, goes on to recount how the *Journal of the American Medical Association* even published an article in 1951 with specific suggestions for what to tell cancer patients, including referring to the cancer as an "ulcer" or an "infection". And its recommendation for any patient who reacted badly to discovering their cancer diagnosis? Lobectomy. However, the work of Dr Elisabeth Kübler-Ross listening to dying patients in Chicago that culminated in her 1969 book *On Death and Dying*,[109] the source of the famous (but now outdated) five stages of grief model, helped to shift the culture around these issues. She made the argument that doctors should be prepared to discuss death openly with their patients.

Dr Robert Buckman was an oncologist who studied at the University of Cambridge, burning the candle at both ends to study medicine by day and perform with the *Cambridge Footlights* by night. It was a training that led to a continued double life as a working doctor and a TV comedian on his BBC show *Pink Medicine*, but it was Buckman's third identity, this time as a patient when he was diagnosed with dermatomyositis in 1978, which radically altered his perspective. Through his own experiences of illness, including believing at one stage that his condition was terminal, Buckman realised that he had in fact coped adequately with each setback thrown at him. He concluded that patients were probably much more resilient than the medical profession had ever given them credit for. Issues concerning death and dying did not need to be tiptoed around – most people just wanted their doctors to honestly convey the facts.

This insight was the catalyst for Buckman's research into how doctors communicated with dying patients, which he conducted alongside his oncology career where he was encountering these issues on a daily basis. This work led to the publication of *I Don't Know What to Say: How to Help and Support Someone Who Is Dying*[110] and, in 1992, *How to Break Bad News*, which was the first ever book on the topic. The steps that Buckman described for breaking bad news evolved into the 'SPIKES' framework, which he elaborated in a paper in the *Oncologist* in 2000 with Walter Baile and others.[111] SPIKES has since become the most well-known and widely taught communication tool for breaking bad news and was the one I was using in the conversation with Tess. The key parts of the SPIKES method are shown in Box 5.1.

It may feel slightly mechanistic to try to systematise such delicate conversations, but a structure or framework can be a helpful starting point, especially when we are relatively inexperienced – and when it is 3 am.

BOX 5.1 SPIKES: A SIX-STEP PROTOCOL FOR BREAKING BAD NEWS

SPIKES

Setting

Optimise set-up: Privacy/Family/Nurse/Sit down/Remove distractions.

Perceptions

Ask open questions to discover: Current understanding/Prior updates/Expectations.

Invitation

What, When and How much does the person want to know?

Knowledge

Tell them the bad news. In chunks. Check understanding.

Empathy

Listen. Be present with them. Use silence. Empathise.

Strategy

Summarise things so far. What are the next steps? Work together on the strategy going forwards.

(After Baile and colleagues, 2000.)

The key is to remember that they are just that – frameworks, which do not need to be rigidly followed to the letter. They are like the Pirate's Code, in that they are "more what you'd call guidelines, than actual rules!" We need to listen to and perceive the verbal and non-verbal cues from the person (or people) we are having the discussion with and adapt what we are saying accordingly. We should also remember that it is ok to differentially prioritise some of the SPIKES steps over others, or even to miss a step altogether depending on the context. For example, the step of seeking the patient's "Invitation" to break the bad news makes sense in the setting of clinical oncology (where the SPIKES model was first conceived), but would come across as bizarre if forced into a conversation with family members you have called into hospital in the middle of the night. Of course they want to know what's going on, and more or less right now! In the original SPIKES paper the authors do comment, "Not every episode of breaking bad news will require all of the steps of SPIKES," but this point can sometimes be missed.

Even very new doctors should feel empowered to trust their human kindness and shape their approach to breaking bad news as the situation demands. Yet if we are de-prioritising or skipping some of the steps, we need to be sure that we're doing this to shape the consultation for the patient or family's benefit and not to make it less uncomfortable for us. Baile and colleagues realised that each of the six SPIKES steps are not equal in terms of their difficulty to execute well. They found when they surveyed 500 attendees at the 1998 American Society of Clinical Oncology "Breaking Bad News Symposium" that more than half (52%) thought they would find the empathy step the most difficult. Only 8% thought they would find the empathy step the easiest. I think this rings true with most people's experiences. When you have just delivered what can often be the worst news imaginable, what on earth should you say next? Perhaps the answer is to say less. When we have dropped a bombshell that has destroyed a family's view of their future, we may just need to "sit in the rubble".

Sitting in the Rubble

Some news that we are required to share with our patients is so bad that "bad" doesn't seem to do it justice. A terminal diagnosis or the death of a parent or husband or wife can be earth-shattering and world-changing, such that it can feel impossible to really put ourselves in our patient's shoes, especially for new doctors who (usually being younger) are less likely to have personal experience with this kind of loss. And in any case, each person's trauma and grief is unique. If we can't truly understand what the other person is going though, how should we best support them? Liz Crowe, an Advanced Clinical Social Worker who is an international expert on grief, loss, trauma and bereavement, was asked in a panel discussion, "We want to help people in this (grief) process, so what framework do we apply to that?" "No framework," she replied. "You get used to sitting in the rubble . . . sit in the rubble with people . . . we're not guiding them anywhere, we're staying with them and keeping them safe"[112]. This phrase, "sitting in the rubble" comes from Judith Murray's book *Understanding Loss*[113] and encapsulates so well what is really required of us in these moments. ICU consultant Matt Morgan explains, "Our nature as healthcare experts is to fix, to solve, and to resolve. But some questions will simply hang over us, with no answer to hand or even ever possible"[114].

The palliative care doctor Rachel Clarke wrote in her second book, *Dear Life*,

> I do not know if words exist to comfort a spouse who sees the love of their life sliding away. Perhaps any solace in those moments must be embodied: the physical fact of your presence, sharing the grief in the cord of your own spine.[115]

This idea of conveying empathy via our physical presence, rather than through words, is shared by palliative care consultant Kathryn Mannix in her book *Listen: How to Find the Words for Tender Conversations*, who puts it like this.

> An empathic response offers companionship in their place of suffering and being prepared to witness, validate, and accompany

> their distress. Empathy identifies with suffering and recognises that either there is no way to fix it or that the solutions must belong to the suffering person. Instead of focusing on doing something, empathy offers to be with someone in their suffering. It is feeling with someone.[116]

Using silence well is possibly the key skill that can help us sit in the rubble. It isn't easy – we can feel like we just need to say something, anything! Yet Dr Mannix reminds us in her "Style Guide" for listening well that you can "use simple expressions to show you are still present" while we "let the silence do its work"[117]. The importance of giving the recipient of the bad news enough space is emphasised in one of the alternative breaking bad news frameworks, which was designed specifically for telling a family that their loved one has died and uses the mnemonic "GRIEV_ING" (Box 5.2). In GRIEV_ING, the underscore represents the essential step of giving the family space to process and digest the information. The original GRIEV_ING study of 20 residents found that learning the framework increased their confidence and competence in conducting death notification conversations,[118] a finding that has since been replicated in fourth-year medical students[119] and in paramedics.[120]

Not attempting to make things better with rushed words in a situation that cannot be fixed is a sign of maturity. It signals to the patient or their family that we have truly understood the magnitude of the news we have just imparted. Instead, we are standing with them as the doors of their no longer possible futures are closed forever, waiting in the silence and staying so that they find we are still there alongside them when they look up from the floor to face their changed and troubling new world. Telling family members that their loved one has died is such a tender conversation because a common wish in our culture is to have witnessed it first-hand, to have been at the deathbed and present in their loved one's final moments. Many people wish to be there at the end.

BOX 5.2 GRIEV_ING: A FRAMEWORK FOR DEATH NOTIFICATION CONVERSATIONS

GRIEV_ING

Gather

The family, in a suitable location

Resources

Human ones for support: Nurse/Chaplain/Second doctor

Identify

Yourself. Them. How much they already know.

Educate

Recap events to date. Educate them about the situation.

Verify

That their loved one has died. Use the 'D' word.
Leave space. Use silence. Let it sink in.

Inquire

Do they have questions? Be prepared to say "I don't know" and refer them to seniors.

Nuts & Bolts

Logistics and practicalities. Viewing the body/Personal belongings/ Death certificate.

Give

Bereavement leaflet. The consultant's secretary's details, in case they have questions later.

(After Hobgood and colleagues, 2005.)

To Be There at the End

When I had been qualified only around six months, back at the Small Hospital, I went to see an elderly woman called Wilma at around 4 am. It was clear that she was desperately unwell. She had been in hospital for weeks and most recently had gone from antibiotic to antibiotic attempting to treat a non-resolving hospital-acquired pneumonia. Yet when I listened to her chest there was no one-sided patch of crackles to find, only wet secretions gurgling everywhere. Her breathing seemed laboured and uneasy. She was deeply unconscious, with no reason to be. I thought that Wilma was dying. She already had a "Do Not Attempt Resuscitation" form in her notes. I discussed things with her staff nurse Louise and we agreed that starting new treatments wasn't appropriate. I prescribed medications for symptom control and wrote all this in her notes. I was sure that she was dying, but I hadn't realised quite how close she was to the end. Perhaps it was that normalcy bias of the night shift's witching hour, that tendency to assume things will play out how you envision, or maybe I was falsely reassured that Louise, too, did not think the end was imminent. I imagined that we would alleviate Wilma's symptoms, she would become settled and peaceful, dawn would break, the day team would arrive, Wilma's family would come to the Small Hospital and she would die surrounded by her loved ones. I imagined this and I did not call Wilma's daughter at 4.30 am. I did not ask my registrar to come and see Wilma. By 7.30 am Wilma had died, with only the half-deflated silver helium balloon from her 95th birthday at her bedside. I was wracked with guilt and still count this among my most troubling mistakes.

In *Listen*, Kathryn Mannix tells a similar story from when she was the most junior doctor in the hospital.[121]

> "Am I dying, doctor?" she was asked.
>
> *I have never been asked this question before. Really? Or have I just never heard it so clearly before. I don't know what to say. She*

is sick enough to die, but she may pull through. It's not my role to discuss this. She should talk to the team she knows, tomorrow.

"Of course not," she heard herself say.

By Monday morning she is dead. She never got to say goodbye to her husband. She didn't have a last cuddle with her daughters. She was asking me for a truth I found too bitter to acknowledge and I lied to her. I may never recover from this shame. Obviously I tell no-one. More than thirty years later, that shame and guilt are as fresh as ever.

It matters so much, beyond rationality or reason, for families to have the opportunity to be with their loved ones in their final days and hours. I learned, through my failure, that this is one of the keystone parts of what it means to keep dying patients safe. President Barack Obama reflected in *A Promised Land* on his guilt and personal struggles with not having been present at his mother's deathbed. "The unspoken regrets. Passing a healthcare bill wouldn't bring my Mom back. It wouldn't douse the guilt I still felt for not having been at her side when she took her last breath"[122]. People, from those of the humblest backgrounds to a President of the United States of America, have these basic human thoughts and worries in common. The desire to be alongside those we love as they die is an instinct, a compulsion born from our love, and when that need is blockaded and barricaded it can feel like a great wrong is being committed.

During Covid-19, with hospital visiting policies varying up and down the UK, this was the scenario that thousands found themselves in, stuck at home in isolation as their loved ones died on hospital wards, feeling alone, with overwhelmed staff hidden behind layers of PPE that lengthened the distance between the care givers and the cared for. The staff nevertheless did all they could to go some way towards putting these wrongs to right.

Early in the Covid-ICU aboard the University Spaceship in 2020, we were caring for Paul, a 58-year-old father of three who had deteriorated despite days of intensive care and was not going to survive. We had tried everything: he had been proned multiple times, we had diagnosed and treated a concurrent pulmonary embolism and super-added ventilator-acquired pneumonia, his kidneys were being supported by a renal filter machine and the ventilator settings had been optimised. Yet he continued to get sicker, despite it all, sporadically flicking into dysrhythmias that threatened cardiac arrest. Paul was going to die. The hospital policy stated that once end-of-life care was initiated, patients could have two visitors, provided they wore full PPE and accepted the risks of entering the ICU. All three of Paul's children were in the waiting area outside. "Well forget this," declared Steve, the ICU charge nurse. "Damn the policy. I'm not making them choose which of them doesn't get to see their Dad." I already held Steve in high esteem, but now I admired him all the more. We dressed Paul's family in the alien attire of the PPE, brought them inside, and they held his hand.

The next week, on the night shift now as we flipped between blocks of four days and four nights, there was a 79-year-old woman called Hilda who also had severe Covid pneumonitis. She too was dying on the ventilator. Reading the notes, it seemed that it had been borderline whether to intubate her, but she had wanted to go ahead, understanding fully that she was more likely than not to die anyhow. And dying she was, her lungs failing despite 100% oxygen supplementation and increasing ventilator pressures. Her family had been forced to make the nightmarish decision not to risk coming into the ICU due to their own health conditions, but one of the consultants, Pietru, promised them over the phone that he would ensure she was cared for and would not be alone. The organ support was withdrawn and Hilda was kept comfortable with one final infusion of medication, yet she did not die as quickly as everyone had expected. With Pietru holding her hand, Hilda stayed with us. The blood pressure reading from the arterial line remained around 40/20 mmHg and Hilda stayed. As the minutes passed, a small collection of us lingered at a distance, witnessing this last act of kindness from a doctor devoted to his patient and the promise he had made to her family. This, surely, was what poet and Covid-ICU survivor Michael Rosen was referring to in the title of his memoir, *Many Different Kinds of Love.*[123] Still Hilda stayed. Eventually, Pietru turned to us and said simply, "I think I'm going to need a chair." A chair was fetched. Pietru sat down and he stayed with Hilda until the end, head bowed and silent in the stillness.

Bearing witness to the deaths of our patients is part of being a doctor and may even be a bigger part of the job for junior doctors, who spend a larger proportion of their time on the wards than their seniors. This role though, as our patients' final doctor, can be an occupational hazard. When we have been looking after patients who are dying or have died, we also need to look after ourselves.

Self-Care

Doctors enjoy the benefits of a highly regarded and esteemed profession, occupying a societal position – and perhaps consequently a psychological position too – with an illusion of superiority. Or should we say delusion. "Patients are patients," we are at risk of thinking. "But we're not like them . . . we're doctors!" Yet of course we are made of the same mortal flesh and blood as those we seek to diagnose and treat, and we feel with the same hearts. It can sometimes seem as though we *should* be able to remain unaffected by the death and trauma we are exposed to, but we cannot be. Doctors deploy all sorts of defence mechanisms to feign ambivalence, but the truth is that it is normal to have feelings about and to react to events that are totally abnormal. It is just that medicine has only very recently begun to acknowledge this reality. We need to give ourselves permission to feel.

Death, in and of itself, is normal – and people often talk about a 'good' death, dying with comfort and dignity and surrounded by loved ones. But when might we find the death of a patient particularly difficult? First asking ourselves what is normal and what is not normal, as related to our existing experience, can be a helpful place to start. For a medical student who has never witnessed a patient die before, even the stereotypical scene of a 'good' death will be highly salient and abnormal. They might wish to talk about the case, what had caused this frail elderly gentleman in Bay 7 to die, and what the next steps would be for his family members. Over time, as they qualify and then begin life on the wards, similar scenarios will become normal, and will even become cases where they reflect positively on their work at the end of the patient's life, derive valuable job satisfaction and have very few, if any, troubling emotions to process afterwards. Notwithstanding this natural progression to becoming more comfortable working side by side with death, there remain several factors that, if present, are likely to make a death more challenging to cope with (Box 5.3). Or equally, there could be no discernible reason at all to feel particularly affected – some things are just so. Either way, we need to have strategies to care for ourselves when we have been a patient's final doctor.

NHS Education for Scotland suggests the mnemonic 'TALK' for helping us cope with death and bereavement as a health or social care professional (Box 5.4).[124] For me, the two key ideas it contains are the fact that "a problem shared is a problem halved" and the need for self-kindness. Both can sometimes be easier said than done. It may not be straightforward to find a suitable time, location and colleague to

BOX 5.3 RISK FACTORS FOR INCREASED DIFFICULTY PROCESSING THE DEATH OF A PATIENT

WHEN MIGHT A PATIENT'S DEATH BE MORE DIFFICULT?

- The death was sudden/unexpected/traumatic
- A child or infant has died
- No DNACPR form, with inappropriate resuscitation attempts
- End-of-life care was sub-optimal
- The case triggers personal memories

BOX 5.4 THE TELL, ASK, LISTEN, KINDNESS MNEMONIC FROM NHS EDUCATION FOR SCOTLAND

TALK

Tell – someone about how you are feeling
Ask – for help and support
Listen – to colleagues, and check how they are doing
Kindness – for yourself and for others

discuss things with after a patient has died. And I have picked out the part about self-kindness because most doctors have no problem with prioritising kindness for others but are not very good at being kind to themselves. Although sections of Jordan B Peterson's *12 Rules for Life* are quite problematic, we would all do well to remember his instruction in "Rule 2" to "Treat yourself like someone you are responsible for helping"[125].

When a patient we are caring for has died, self-kindness is important in the longer term but also in the immediate aftermath of the event. We have already seen the benefits of taking short breaks (or even micro-breaks if that is all time will allow) on the night shift, and here too breaks can be vital, helping us to emotionally reset before continuing with the rest of the shift's work. Professor Roger Neighbour coined the term 'housekeeping' in *The Inner Consultation*[126] to describe how GPs should acknowledge and process the immediate emotions arising from a consultation before seeing the next patient in the clinic. We may need to pause for some housekeeping in the hospital too. What we do in this short pause is a personal choice – it could be a walk (ideally outside) for a few minutes, a coffee, some music or even a short meditation from an app on our phone. What is important is that we do something to be kind to ourselves.

One particularly interesting tactic suggested by Neighbour is combining the use of an 'icon' with a psychological technique called 'anchoring' that comes from the field of neuro-linguistic programming. If you're thinking that this sounds a bit voodoo, hear it out. The icon can be any designated object that is associated with personal wellbeing, for example a keyring in your scrub pocket from a favourite holiday, a photo from the natural world on your iPhone or even a potted plant on your desk. Simply having the icon with you or near you to look at is a good thing, but its power can be supercharged by anchoring it to a positive visualisation where you were at (or close to) your most relaxed and happy. Close your eyes. Take yourself back to that place, that time, with the sights and smells and sounds that were present and focus on how calm and content you had been there. The more detail you can recall, the more layers of paint you put on the canvas, the stronger it will be. Stay in that visualisation for as long as you can, until it is as complete as you can make it. When you're ready, open your eyes, come back to the present moment and then stare at your icon, whilst at the same time squeezing your left thumb with your right hand. Repeat this a couple of times to reinforce the brain circuitry you're wiring up. "You can now use either the icon or the grip of the thumb", writes Neighbour, "whenever you need an infusion of tranquillity."

However, in certain rarer cases the strategies discussed so far may feel as though they will not be anything like enough to help us. What should our approach be if we have witnessed a death that is so incredibly traumatic and shocking that we have no idea where even to begin in processing the resulting emotional and psychological distress?

Matt Walton was a final year medical student on an elective placement with the Essex & Hertfordshire Air Ambulance when he encountered such a case. On the last flight of his elective, the team were called to a "possible dead child", a warning sign the team perceived as ominous, noting the absence of the more formal term 'paediatric traumatic cardiac arrest'.

"It was much worse than I had imagined," wrote Matt in a *BMJ* opinion piece in 2018.[127] He recalled the "critically ill child in the midst of blue flashing police lights, hysterical onlookers, and hectic activity". Despite receiving world-class pre-hospital care, the child died. "I managed to keep focused and professional," Matt wrote. "But later, the full horror sank in."

Where to begin? In a short YouTube film Matt produced about the incident,[128] the Critical Care paramedic from that day, Tony Stone, explained, "When we got back to base, I felt that it was really important for all of us to sit down and try and debrief this incident. . . . The scene itself was very visually distressing and it was horrible to see." Dr Mike Christian, the team's pre-hospital consultant, added that part of the role of a debrief is "to start the preparations for what might come next, the beginning of that process of getting through these bad jobs".

Recognising the gravity of what he had witnessed and the likelihood that processing the psychological trauma would not be straightforward, before leaving the team base Matt had asked Dr Christian simply, "What do I do now?" Mike Christian presciently explained about some of the things he may face: memories coming back, intrusive thoughts or even flashbacks. "I think one of the most important things is to let people know what normal is, letting them know that's normal and that it gets better over time," he says. This support from a highly experienced consultant went a long way and was invaluable when intrusive thoughts did start coming Matt's way. Matt says, "It would have been quite a scary thing had Mike not told me that was normal, and it wasn't something to be worried about and he experienced it too." Mike Christian also followed up with text messages some weeks later to check how Matt was doing.

Matt Walton draws attention to how rotating medical students "can just slip through the net" and "don't know if what we're experiencing is normal", or know where to seek help. The same can be said for new doctors, who have shorter rotations than their more senior colleagues and may not have accessed formal or informal sources of support, especially if a critical incident occurs at the start of a placement where they remain a relative outsider. We need to create the space for new doctors (and the whole team) to consider their emotional reactions to trauma and death – physical space to sit and reflect, space in the shift with adequate staffing to allow suitable pauses after distressing events, and the psychological space we can open up by talking to someone we trust, asking for advice, listening well and being kind to each other and to ourselves. I realise that we have come full circle and I have just listed the four steps of the 'TALK' mnemonic again. The difference, when we are talking about events that have been incredibly traumatic and totally outside a trainee's bank of experience, is that the burden of responsibility for supporting staff must shift, at least to some degree, towards the formal channels, without losing the support from informal ones. When the magnitude of our psychological shock is likely to be high, we need to do better than a cup of coffee and cracking on. The right place for the British stiff upper lip is in the orange clinical waste bin of history. Some formal sources of support for medical students and doctors are listed in Box 5.5.

In the final section of this chapter, we have considered the importance of caring for ourselves when one of our patients has died. However, paying attention to the effect of our work on our emotions and our wellbeing is a more global endeavour, and indeed some of the coping strategies discussed so far may be helpful outside the specific setting of end-of-life care, death and bereavement. In Chapter 6, we will think more broadly about psychological distress in young doctors, addressing some specific elements of the circumstances new doctors often find themselves in.

Box 5.5 SOME NATIONAL ORGANISATIONS THAT OFFER PSYCHOLOGICAL SUPPORT

PSYCHOLOGICAL SUPPORT FOR DOCTORS

- British Medical Association wellbeing services, including counselling and peer-support – these are open to all medical students and doctors, regardless of BMA membership.
  www.bma.org.uk/advice-and-support/your-wellbeing/wellbeing-support-services/counselling-and-peer-support-services

- DocHealth – a confidential, not for profit, psychotherapeutic consultation service for qualified doctors, supported by the BMA and the Royal Medical Benevolent Fund.
  www.dochealth.org.uk

- The Intensive Care Society wellbeing resources for staff – much of the information these contain will prove useful even for those not working in Intensive Care.
  www.ics.ac.uk/Society/Wellbeing_hub/Resources_for_Staff

"Sassal has made a Faustian pact: he is rewarded with endless opportunities for experiencing the possibilities inherent in human lives, but at the cost of being subject to immense, and at times unbearable pressures."

Gavin Francis, Introduction to
A Fortunate Man: The Story of a Country Doctor
by John Berger and Jean Mohr

"We knew that it could have been any of us. Lethal, this becoming and being a doctor!"

Samuel Shem, *The House of God*

6

CLINGING TO THE RAFT

PSYCHOLOGICAL DISTRESS IN NEW DOCTORS

Physician, Heal Thyself

As we filed into the lecture theatre seats on that Wednesday afternoon, I knew that something was wrong. We were several months into our first year working as doctors and we always had Wednesday afternoons reserved for teaching sessions, but there were more people, and different people, standing at the front of the lecture theatre compared to usual. In addition to the team who worked in the postgraduate office, there was the medical director dressed formally in suit and tie. And, was that the chief executive? Once we had quietened down, coats and bags shoved under our seats, the medical director stepped to the front.

"I'm very sorry to be here before you this afternoon," he began. "Some of you, sadly, will already know what I've come to speak to you about." I did not. I was in the dark. I looked left and right. Some of my colleagues looked equally confused, while others were looking down at the floor. "Two days ago, the Trust became aware of the death of a junior doctor at the hospital accommodation on one of our sites. She was in the second year of the programme. Her death is not being treated as suspicious, and it appears that tragically she took her own life."

The medical director continued speaking, but I had temporarily tuned out. My mind was spinning. I had been aware of the national news coverage surrounding doctors' high levels of stress, burnout and mental health disorders, but this was too close to home. ". . . and please be aware that we have many services available to help, so please do use them if you or anyone you know is struggling," the director was saying. "This number on the screen is my mobile number. You can call me anytime day or night if you need to talk." I remember thinking that calling the medical director would be a difficult step to take, but admiring him for it all the same.

Doctor suicide is what unites the two quotes that preface this chapter, yet they differ in their referring to either intrinsic or extrinsic sources of psychological strain. John Sassal (real surname Eskell) was a rural GP whose life and work was the subject of writer John Berger's and photographer Jean Mohr's 1967 book *A Fortunate Man*.[129] After his wife's death in the early 1980s, Sassal shot himself. GP Gavin Francis, who provided the introduction to the modern reprinted edition of *A Fortunate Man*, alluded to the risks inherent in empathetic doctoring in the *Guardian* when he wrote that Sassal's "openness to experience – his gift to the world – was also his undoing"[130]. The double-edged sword of empathy, intrinsic to the practice of medicine, is something we will return to. The second quote, from *The House of God*, is a reference to the suicide of 'Potts', one of the first-year residents in Samuel Shem's quasi-autobiographical novel about life in a Boston hospital in the 1970s. Unable to cope with the pressures of the system, unsupported by his seniors and wracked with guilt from a fatal early mistake, Potts had jumped from an 8th floor window. The book's protagonist, Roy, reflected, "No-one mentioned how the House Medical Hierarchy had tormented Potts . . . how it had ignored his pain"[131].

Why am I quoting from two books that relate to medical life in the 1960s and 1970s? Because the issue of how our work puts our mental health – and even our lives – at risk, remains as pressing as it has ever been. "House Medical Hierarchy" could today be a metaphor for the medical regulators whose dispassionate or clumsy handling of several high-profile cases of doctors undergoing investigations has been linked to those doctors' subsequent suicides. Whilst suicide is the most shocking manifestation of the strains new doctors can find themselves experiencing, depression and the (related, but distinct) syndrome of burnout have also been at epidemic levels in the profession since well-before Covid-19 worsened the situation substantially. In many ways, it is a frightening era to be becoming a new doctor.

A complete description and analysis of the physician mental health crisis is well beyond the scope of this chapter, but for those who are interested one comprehensive text is Clare Gerada's *Beneath the White Coat: Doctors, Their Minds and Mental Health*.[132] Of course, mental health difficulties don't only affect doctors, and I am convinced that by far the best thing we can do for our mental health is to double down on the same basics we would advise for our patients, which means eating properly, drinking more water, doing some exercise, trying to sleep for 8 hours per night, doing some form of mindfulness or meditation and ideally trying to find someone to talk to as well. These things are incredibly important, but they are already widely discussed and are not specific to new doctors. Therefore, we will examine the psychology behind some of the issues that are particularly relevant for new doctors as we start out in our careers, in the hope that framing and understanding these elements of our professional and our personal lives might offer useful perspectives on how we can better care for ourselves and – by extension – our patients.

One key issue is the way in which the stark contrast between the experiences of our medical work and those of non-medical 'normal life' can give rise to a growing sense of disconnection with those around us. Paradoxically, as the months of successfully completed doctoring post-graduation begin to accumulate and we become more settled in our once ill-fitting and anxiously worn metaphorical white coats, that same subconscious embedding of a new identity can itself cast us further adrift from our previous lives and familiar sources of support. We can begin to find ourselves torn between two worlds.[133]

Between Two Worlds

On one occasion, at this point several months into my first year as a doctor, I had a few days off after a run of night shifts and was away from the city, staying at my grandparents' house. They live in a one-road village that has some houses, a church, a village hall, a cricket pitch, a pub and a red telephone box that now contains a defibrillator rather than a telephone. It is situated in rolling farmland, a location that could be described as either "idyllic and rural" or "in the middle of nowhere", depending on your perspective. Some years before, when the phone box had *not* contained a defibrillator, my Granny (who is a retired nurse) might just for a moment have come down on the side of "in the middle of nowhere" as she single-handedly performed 20 minutes of CPR to save the life of a fellow villager in cardiac arrest, whilst waiting for the ambulance to arrive. Their village was certainly remote and far away from any city, yet my mind was still half in the District General Hospital, preoccupied with the events of the preceding night shifts. Our patients had been desperately unwell. I had worked almost non-stop to dash between those who were scared, in pain, deteriorating and needing reviewing, or dying and needing medication to stave off their suffering. It was not easy to switch off. I was not fully relaxing and enjoying the time away.

My parents were also with us and there was going to be a family gathering for Granny's 81st birthday. As we sat around that morning, waiting for people to arrive, my brother and my Mum (who are both teachers) were discussing their workloads and what sounded like very silly staffroom politics at their respective schools. Their debate continued, but it all sounded so arbitrary, I thought angrily. Did it even matter? What did they have to worry about anyhow? Eventually, I had heard enough and said abruptly, "Is it really such a problem? It's not like anyone died!" There was a moment of shocked silence in the room. I had lost my composure, and they did not know what to say. How could they?

The problem I was encountering, I can see now, is one that was definitely not unique to me, or indeed to doctors in general, but rather is endemic in the caring professions, from social work to nursing to medicine to midwifery. In *The Language of Kindness*, Christie Watson writes,

> I find that my friends are all becoming doctors, nurses and midwives, and my non-nursing friends are dropping off. One who works in an office complains all the time about her difficult day. Another complains that his baby's crying is worrying him so much, there might be something wrong. 'Really sick babies don't cry,' I say. I have decreasing sympathy for normal problems. Friends I grew up with ask about nursing. 'It's hard to explain,' I tell them. 'You are changing,' they tell me.[134]

In the same way that Christie Watson was finding it easier to maintain friendships with colleagues with whom she retained a lot of shared experience, I was similarly finding it difficult to empathise with my family's day-to-day work dilemmas and to honestly answer my university friends when they asked me how the job was going. Where could I even start?

The simple truth is that the gritty and unglamorous work of doctoring, bearing witness on an almost daily basis to the intense moments of physical or emotional distress that most people experience on only a few occasions in their lives, does not make for good dinner party conversation. Or cocktail party conversation. Or good conversation for a grandparent's birthday party. Instead, we tend to default to short, well-rehearsed, easily contained anecdotes that win us an expected laugh and deflect from how we're really doing. We reel off our playbook, the material either our own or borrowed from colleagues: ". . . and the toothbrush she had swallowed showed up on the chest X-ray! Who knew that plastic bristles would be radio-opaque?" or "He was adamant that he had fallen awkwardly and *landed* on the TV remote . . . I thought about asking if it had turned him on, but that seemed unprofessional so I kept a straight face and referred him to colorectal!" Alternatively, we might make generalised comments about the state of the NHS. "Well, there were 17 ambulances queued up outside A&E when I left yesterday evening, but that's about normal," we'll say, shifting the conversation onto familiar ground and once more avoiding the original topic of how we're doing. This is our usual modus operandi, these conversational sleights of hand subconsciously deployed to bridge what can feel like an impassable divide between our two worlds. In my outburst at my grandparents' house, I had broken the rules, signalling my mounting fatigue and underlying distress.

In fact, rather than knowingly breaking what can seem like unwritten rules, what I had failed to manage was something called 'cultural code-switching', an idea that may be central to navigating a path within and between our medical and non-medical worlds. Narrow definitions of cultural code-switching have been purely linguistic, defining it as "changing from one way of speaking to another between or within interactions" and including "changes in accent, dialect or language"[135]. Using the right language with the right people is definitely applicable to the switch required between our medical and our home lives – we could not talk about witnessing a rapid sequence induction prior to clamshell thoracotomy for pericardial tamponade at the dinner table and expect anyone to understand what on earth we were on about. However, broader conceptions of cultural code-switching that include the need to suppress aspects of our cultural identity[136] and switch between potentially conflicting value systems[137] get closer to what is required of doctors. Cultural code-switching between the medical and non-medical worlds could be thought of as the shift required of healthcare staff to match that culture's language, frames of reference, value system, expectations and interpersonal understanding of previous experiences. This definition suggests that if we are speaking about that thoracotomy at dinner we have probably failed to code-switch altogether.

Being able to adeptly code-switch is, I think, an important part of protecting our mental wellbeing as new doctors. It is much easier said than done, and if there is a skill to be mastered here then I remain far from mastering it. And, at first, the whole idea can seem disingenuous or even duplicitous. Why should we have to constantly switch between two versions of ourselves, versions that have been formed in two staggeringly different worlds? Isn't suppressing distress arising in our medical world exactly the wrong way to look after our mental health? Of course, it would be, if it were to be suppressed altogether. To successfully code-switch, we need to have adequate psychosocial support embedded within our medical world, whether that arrives via informal networks of friends and colleagues, or via more formalised support services promoted and funded by our institutions. Only when we are adequately supported to manage work-induced psychological distress will we retain enough emotional capital to repeatedly and successfully make the transition between the two worlds.

Doctors' ability to code-switch is both a causative factor and a symptom when it comes to our mental wellbeing. If we lose the ability to code-switch, our disconnection from our home (non-medical) world containing our significant others and previously dependable sources of support will increase, making us more vulnerable to loneliness, burnout and mental illness. This is code-switching (or the lack of it) as aetiology. But equally, when we are not mentally present in our home world and not fully benefiting from what should be restorative time away from work, with or without overt demonstrations of unresolved psychological distress like my outburst at my grandparents', this is failed code-switching as symptomatology, showing that all is not well.

It seems, then, that learning to understand and successfully navigate our new and evolving identities as doctors in an often-distressing medical world depends primarily on the way in which that psychological distress is processed. Can we detach ourselves from it? Should we detach ourselves from it? Are we not required to be empathetic practitioners, trying to put ourselves in our patients' shoes to understand what they are going through? I first became interested in these questions as a medical student back in 2016, researching and writing about the tension that exists between our aspirations for empathy and a drive for detachment that has been transmitted down the medical generations. The following section is an adaptation and extension of an article I wrote in the *British Journal of General Practice* titled "Increasing Emotional Support for Healthcare Workers Can Rebalance Clinical Detachment and Empathy"[138].

The Detachment Doctrine

As healthcare professionals we are confronted with patients' emotional traumas on a daily, if not hourly basis. Faced with this kind of distress, we might exhibit (and experience) what I will call 'true empathy'. This kind of empathy involves feeling another's emotions oneself as an 'emotional resonance', rather than just correctly acknowledging them.[139] Alternatively, we may exercise 'clinical detachment', a conscious choice to numb ourselves to emotional resonance with our patients in order to maintain scientific objectivity, and to help us cope, to carry on for the benefit of the next patient in line. Although true empathy and clinical detachment must be mutually exclusive in their purest forms, the choice between them is a false dichotomy. For the majority of clinicians, their response to emotional trauma will lie somewhere between the two, held in an uncomfortable equilibrium governed by cultural or institutional belief systems and competing doctor and patient agendas. At their extremes, true empathy and clinical detachment hold potential for unintended progression to emotional exhaustion or a generalised emotional detachment, respectively, both viewed as components of burnout. Therefore, the ideal response to emotional trauma might be an exact balance between true empathy and clinical detachment, minimising the risks associated with either extreme, while retaining some of the benefits of each approach. Unfortunately, medicine has long been heavily skewed towards clinical detachment.

Ever since William Hunter, an 18th century surgeon–anatomist, suggested that his students should acquire "a necessary inhumanity" through dissection,[140] an acceptance of clinical detachment as the appropriate disposition has become pervasive. Sir William Osler wrote in his 1912 essay *Aequanimitas*,[141] "A rare and precious gift is the art of detachment" and argued that doctors might objectively "see into" a patient's "inner life" by neutralising their emotions to the point that they feel nothing in response to suffering. Further, Hunter's original view of the dissection room as a training ground for developing clinical detachment has persisted into the 21st century. Hildebrandt notes that the finding that medical students at Ulm University reported decreased empathy as their dissection course progressed[142] may in fact represent their having acquired the trait of clinical detachment.[143]

The realities of today's clinical arena similarly drive us towards clinical detachment as the default. Rapid scientific progress has produced modern diagnostic and therapeutic options that are steeped in technical data and challenging procedures, all of which need to be managed by clear-thinking clinician scientists. Now more than ever, the idea of clinical detachment as a prerequisite for scientific objectivity[144] will ring true for health workers. This mindset may also be reinforced by the immense workloads, time pressures, and target-driven cultures of many health systems, factors that would make clinicians more likely to choose the short-term coping benefits of detachment over the patient-centred benefits of true empathy.

Contending with the Covid-19 pandemic at the start of the first wave in March 2020 brought the issue of clinical detachment into sharp relief. At first, I tried to imagine the experiences of the patients we were caring for. I tried to imagine what it must be like, struggling to breathe, working hard, gasping for breath despite the strongest oxygen mask the hospital can give you, coping, treading water at the surface but knowing that you cannot carry on without relent. The ICU consultant arriving, explaining that to have any chance of surviving you would have to be put to sleep and attached to a ventilator, and that even in this case they thought that there was approximately a 50% chance you would never wake up. Then they would leave, tidal waves rather than ripples extending in all directions around the stone they had cast. Some time. Not enough time. Time to Facetime one, or two or three of the people you loved most in all the world, raising your voice to be heard above the hissing high-flow oxygen that is holding your space here, for now, for the moment, for a little longer.

And then the time comes and the anaesthetics consultant arrives, accompanied by their team, which is comprised of the fewest possible number of people, in order to minimise exposure, exposure to the risk of you. They're talking now, explaining things, slowly, caringly, but you're not really hearing and the time is speeding up. "We're just setting up a few more things to monitor you, to keep you safe. . . . We're going to look after you." More preparing, more arranging of equipment. They tell you how the next stage will be for them to put you off to sleep, before inserting the breathing tube that will attach you to the ventilator. And the ventilator will attach you to this world. Things are ready now, they tell you to think about someplace sunny, and you fill your mind with images born far away from here. You focus on them, rather than what is coming. Your eyes are closed now, and you suddenly feel a little sleepy. A half-formed image of someone you used to know appears for a moment, but they seem somehow distant . . . and then you are gone.

I didn't carry on thinking about it for very long. I couldn't have. As the ICU filled up with patient after patient wheeled onto the unit from an intubation room, exiting a scene like the one I had tried to imagine, the patients were already dehumanised and depersonalised by their attachment to their machines, as we were by the gowns and masks and visors we wore. So many patients of a similar age and medical background, with the same diagnosis, needing the same management, meant that it was feeling like a production line. I had to focus in order to avoid mixing the patients up, such was their uniformity. I only prescribed their medicines whilst stood at the computer at the foot of their bed, to reduce the chances of making an error. Even when I called their families back home, people waiting in terror for what the day's update might bring, I was not emotionally engaged.

> He's still needing high amounts of oxygen provided through the ventilator and still needing the kidney machine to do their job of filtering the blood. He remains critically unwell. I'm so sorry it's not the news you've been hoping for, but there's been very little change and we don't know which way things are going to go.

We did the best we could, tried to be the kindest we could, but with the need to carry on for week after week after week, it was, overall, a case of clinical detachment par excellence.

With or without Covid, when we lack the tools to interpret troubling emotions, or we do not believe ourselves capable of doing so, we opt instead for a predominantly detached response. "I'd stare at my colleagues and wonder about everything we weren't discussing," writes Dr Rana Awdish in her memoir *In Shock: How Nearly Dying Made Me a Better Intensive Care Doctor*.[145]

> How it felt to be responsible for a bad outcome. How it felt to make such an awful disclosure to the family. How it felt to round on the patient day after day, confronted by the concrete aftermath of your choices. It seemed a terrible blind spot that we did not

> discuss the toll those errors exacted on us. . . . We have utterly no idea what to do with shame. We have built no confessionals.

This feeling of an inability to process emotional resonance, alongside the lack of institutional structures designed to help us do so, is arguably the most important driver of our over-detachment because it is the most amenable to change. Dr Awdish has since become a national and international campaigner for improving empathy and the patient experience, alongside training faculty and trainees in relationship-based communication skills.[146] By promoting strategies to better interpret emotional resonance arising from medicine's traumas, we can provide a buffer, facilitating a shift back towards a balance between true empathy and clinical detachment.

One promising way of supporting healthcare staff is the implementation of Schwartz Center Rounds®, monthly multidisciplinary meetings focused on discussing the emotional and social aspects of healthcare work. These one-hour sessions involve the presentation of a case study and discussion of the emotional issues it raised, followed by time for questions, reflection and the sharing of similar experiences, led by a trained facilitator. A 2012 qualitative analysis of the rounds in two UK pilot sites suggested that rounds increased respect, understanding and empathy between staff,[147] a benefit that consultant psychologist Leslie Morrison said was beginning to be shown to "spill over into a greater sense of compassion and empathy for patients". Since then, the first large-scale evaluation of Schwartz Center Rounds in the UK has found that regular attenders at rounds developed significantly fewer minor psychiatric disorders (evaluated using the GHQ-12 questionnaire) when compared with a control group of non-attenders.[148] The study's authors conclude that whilst "providing high-quality health care has an emotional impact on staff" and they "experience high levels of psychological distress", the safe space offered by the Schwartz Rounds forum has improved attendees' practice and facilitated an increase in their empathy for colleagues and patients alike.

Promoting clinical empathy with interventions such as Schwartz Rounds is so important because, despite the short-term benefits, the long-term harms of detachment can be profound. In her bestselling book *Daring Greatly*, Professor Brené Brown argues, "We can't selectively numb emotion. Numb the dark and you numb the light"[149]. I had therefore concluded my 2016 article by arguing that systems level change to provide better emotional support for healthcare workers could offer the foundations for a shift towards true empathy, and away from clinical detachment. I was advocating for changes that might lead to a shift in our set-point on that spectrum, helping us to reach some kind of Goldilocks zone where we could have the benefits, but avoid the harms, of both dispositions. The reality, of course, is a little more complicated.

As I progressed in my clinical training and then started working as a doctor, I learned how we need to be able to be truly empathetic in some moments, and clinically detached at others. A good example would be doctors such as the paediatric neurosurgeon Jay Jayamohan, who we heard from in Chapter 3. The parents of the small children on whom he operates need him to be kind and empathetic at the moment he breaks the news of their child's brain tumour, but ruthlessly focused and detached from the point that he scrubs up to operate and remove it. Back on the wards, now in my fourth year since qualification at the time of writing, when I stand at the end of the bed and lead the cardiac arrest team there is no room for empathy for the family I know the patient has at home. I am only thinking about the algorithm, the team, the lifeless patient before us and a detached consideration of the physiology.

Although it has taken the ensuing years of clinical training for me to fully appreciate it, this more nuanced view of the need for clinicians to display both dispositions and minimise psychological distress by honing the skill of switching between the two was in fact swiftly pointed out to me in a published reply to my article from Roger Neighbour.[150] Roger is a retired GP who was propelled to fame amongst GPs nationwide (and later worldwide) by his 1987 book *The Inner Consultation*, in which he elaborated a five-step structure for the medical consultation and coined the term 'safety-netting'[151]. You will recall that we came across *The Inner Consultation* in the previous chapter when discussing 'housekeeping'. In his letter, Roger wrote,

> Sooner or later – and it's often while at medical school – all doctors experience situations that are unforgettably shocking or traumatic. Many of us respond self-protectively by detaching our human responses in order to cope. It's as if a switch is thrown, disconnecting our clinical skills from our emotional intelligence.

In a central chapter of his 2016 book *The Inner Physician*, Roger called this "Crichton's switch", named after the late Michael Crichton (of *Jurassic Park* fame) who had described experiencing this sort of mental "click" in the dissection room at Harvard Medical School when faced with the task of neatly cutting a human head into two halves down the midline.[152] Crichton, too, envisioned an optimal set point between empathy and detachment, writing, "the best doctors found a middle position where they were neither overwhelmed by their feelings nor estranged from them"[153]. However, keeping with Crichton's metaphor of a mental switch, Roger went on to explain why being washed up halfway between these two dispositions, neither fully one nor the other, isn't the best way to look at the problem. He quoted the novelist EM Forster in *Howards End* who wrote,

> The businessman who assumes that this life is everything, and the mystic who asserts that it is nothing, fail to hit the truth. No; truth, being alive, was not halfway between anything. It was only to be found by continuous excursions into either realm.[154]

He concluded with the advice for new doctors (or medical students as I was at the time): "The professional skill, if there is one, is to be in control of it (Crichton's switch), able to engage or disengage our empathy according to clinical circumstances."

Roger's letter was the start of a correspondence that went on to become one of the most trusted friendships in my late university and early professional life. I have been lucky to have him as a mentor and friend, such is his skill in patiently listening and somehow always asking the one or two questions that get straight to what matters. I can't help but think that all new doctors could use a friend like Roger. One of the recurring themes in my conversations with him has been the feeling of being unable to care for patients to the standards we were trained to, due to system failures, time constraints, sheer volume overload or otherwise. I know now that this feeling has been well described and has a name. It is called 'moral distress', which, left unchecked, can progress to 'moral injury'.

Moral Distress

Moral distress can be defined as "the psychological unease generated when professionals identify an ethically correct action to take but are constrained in their ability to take that action" or "the feeling of unease stemming from situations where institutionally required behaviour does not align with moral principles"[155]. Importantly, it is also possible to experience what I would regard as 'bystander moral distress' arising from "witnessing moral transgressions by others". Moral injury can occur when the repeated experiencing of moral distress leads to longer-term psychological harm, which may include diagnosable mental health disorders such as depression and PTSD. Possibly the most important factor driving moral distress is the institutional resource constraints healthcare workers face on a daily basis, which may be human resources (understaffing), space (particularly bed availability), equipment or the time needed to offer compassionate care. A simple illustration of suggested causative factors and the relationship between moral distress, moral injury and adverse psychiatric outcomes is shown in Figure 6.1.

The 2021 BMA report that provided the preceding definitions of moral distress also included the first "pan-profession" survey focused

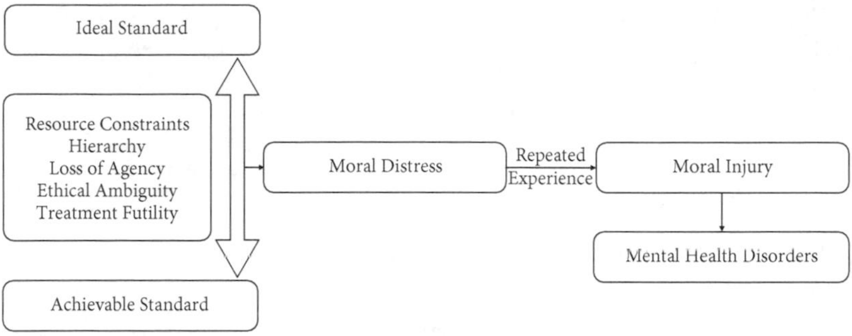

Figure 6.1 Moral distress. A perceived discrepancy between the ideal standard of care (according to formal training, national or local standards, or personal values) and the achievable standard of care can lead to moral distress amongst healthcare staff. Repeatedly experiencing moral distress over the longer term can lead to moral injury, which is associated with increased risk of mental health disorders such as depression and PTSD.

on moral distress and moral injury, conducted between March and April 2021, after the 1st and 2nd waves of the Covid-19 pandemic. Of 1900 survey respondents, 78.4% said that moral distress resonated with their experiences at work and 51.1% said this about moral injury. During the peaks of the Covid-19 pandemic, the overwhelming surge in patient numbers and the widespread experience of families not being permitted to visit dying relatives certainly worsened moral distress and moral injury among healthcare workers. I also think that the cognitive dissonance arising from the disparity between media portrayals of staff as 'NHS Heroes' and our feeling that the care we were providing was sub-standard was another contributor to our collective moral distress.

However, it is clear that moral distress was a pressing issue well before SARS-CoV-2 ever existed. When specifically asked, 59.6% of those surveyed reported experiencing moral distress in the 12 months before the pandemic. One strong memory I have of experiencing what

I would now recognise as moral distress occurred in the pre-Covid era. Amit was a gentleman in his mid-70s suffering from a nasty haematological malignancy, who was referred to ICU in the middle of the night. It appeared that he was heading into multi-organ failure. Realising that his time was short, he had told my registrar that he wanted to get home to be with his family, and the notes from that consultation said as much. Nobody from the ICU team was optimistic that Amit would survive this episode, but the haematologists and oncologists seemed to think that they had one more drug that could give him a chance. Despite what Amit had said about wanting to go home, somehow he had ended up agreeing to come down to the ICU and be put to sleep on the ventilator. "I don't understand why we're doing this," his ICU nurse said to me quietly. "Me neither," I replied. I had heard the phrase "hospital politics" mentioned somewhere along the way, and I didn't like it one bit. Amit died on the ventilator less than two days later. ICU nurses are thought to be particularly vulnerable to moral distress,[156] perhaps because of their role in enacting difficult ethical decisions that have ultimately been made by others. New doctors, too, are especially vulnerable, albeit for slightly different reasons.

The BMA's 2021 survey found that 88.5% of foundation-year doctors recognised moral distress as resonating with their experiences at work, which was significantly higher than the survey's respondents in general (78.4%). It makes sense theoretically that moral distress is likely to be more prevalent amongst doctors at the start of their careers because the comparatively short time elapsed since their training delineating the ideal standards of patient care means they will be more likely to instinctively recognise a disparity between that standard and what they feel the system is allowing them to provide. In her memoir *Breaking & Mending*, Joanna Cannon describes this disillusionment and disconnect when she writes,

> All the way through medical school, the one thing that keeps you going . . . is the idea of what kind of doctor you are going

> to be. . . . It's only when you arrive on the wards, when you are spat out into an NHS that bends and breaks under the strain of endless demands placed upon it, it's only then that you realise you will never be able to be the doctor you want to become. The system simply won't allow it.[157]

The internal conflict new doctors experience as they wonder whether their difficulties in providing what they would regard as good care are stemming from their own beginner status and lack of clinical experience could also contribute to the feeling of moral distress. In Chapter 3 we heard Sanith describe the early weeks on the wards as "battling your own sense of self-efficacy", adding that "feeling rubbish, like you can't do something, really affects your self-confidence". For those new doctors who are slower to appreciate that it is usually a multitude of adverse systems factors rather than the individual that is responsible for sub-optimal care, the feeling that personal inadequacies are to blame will very likely become injurious. Finally, new doctors in their position at the bottom of the hierarchy are more vulnerable to feelings of lacking power or agency, not feeling supported in decision-making, or feeling as though they should be challenging questionable end-of-life decision-making from senior doctors, all of which may trigger moral distress.

What can we do about it? Any definitive solutions will require systems-based change at the level of government and our institutions to tackle the constraints that stop us doing the job we were trained to do. We can and should be unionised and keep campaigning for decisive change, however far away that may feel as we tread water in the era of Covid-19. Because moral distress can be triggered by task overload, difficult decision-making, things going wrong, cultures that discourage speaking up, work-related fatigue and tricky end-of-life care issues, it is an issue that unifies aspects of every preceding chapter so far. Incremental improvements in the way that new doctors are supported in each of these areas should, therefore, have a knock-on effect on moral distress. In the meantime, it is all we can do to keep on looking after ourselves and each other. We need these close and supportive relationships at work, but they can be hard to lose.

The Price of Goodbye

Another source of psychological strain that is particularly relevant to young doctors is the burden imposed by the frequent formation of, and then loss of, high value working relationships. In the UK, new doctors switch jobs every four months for their first two years, sometimes changing not only department and specialty, but town and hospital too. Although plenty of young professionals undertake similar programmes of rotations at the start of their careers (newly qualified lawyers starting out in large firms or civil servants moving through various government departments spring to mind), the nature of medical work means that the relationships we form can be especially intense and meaningful, despite the relatively short length of time they have existed.

The novelist Francesca Segal captured this tendency for the medical world to create interpersonal bonds at unparalleled pace in her memoir *Mother Ship*, an account of the weeks she spent at a major hospital with her newly born twins struggling for their lives in the Neonatal ICU. Describing the growing friendship between herself and one of the other mothers there, she wrote,

> We are allowing each other to spill into the remaining sliver of our lives outside the NICU and, as with space, so with time. We met three and a half weeks ago, but what is now between us was forged in the frontier's white heat. In this, my new life, I have known her life-long.[158]

What is true for families and patients is also true for clinicians, since we are all only humans, confronting some of the extremes of human experience. In *When Breath Becomes Air*, the late Paul Kalanithi wrote, "Drowning, even in blood, one adapts, learns to float, to swim, even to enjoy life, bonding with the nurses, doctors, others who are clinging to the same raft, caught in the same tide"[159]. Therefore, when we lose the ones we have been working with for many weeks and months, the people we have forged connections with that should, by rights, have taken years to develop, it can feel like a heavy loss to endure.

Why is it that these frequent rotations can take such a toll? Is it not the case that they offer us the chance to accumulate more and more of these meaningful connections in our early working lives, which has to be a good thing, doesn't it? The answers might be found in evolutionary anthropology, a discipline that has suggested an explanation for why, when it comes to social connections, losses are an inevitability. In the early 1990s, anthropologist Robin Dunbar published his research into the relationship between the sizes of the neocortices of various primates and their average social group size.[160] After a clear ratio between these variables emerged, Dunbar's eureka moment arrived when he realised that he could apply that ratio to the neocortical volume of *Homo sapiens* to produce an estimate for the expected human social group size. It turned out to be around 150. To put this number to the test, Dunbar's team looked at traditional hunter–gatherer communities still living today much as they would have done thousands of years ago. Their typical group size was indeed around 150. Furthermore, the average village size in the Doomsday book was 150, and parish registers from multiple UK counties in the 18th century (before the industrial revolution dramatically changed the distribution of citizens across British settlements) also showed an average village size of 150. This 'magic number' of 150 has become known as 'Dunbar's number'.

Nowadays, in modern societies where we live in large cities and towns and even single apartment blocks that are home to well over 150 people, Dunbar's number no longer describes the size of the group with whom we share physical proximity. Yet in today's world it still represents the limits of our close social connections. When you account for multiple people living within one household, most people's Christmas card lists mean sending greetings to approximately 150 friends.[161] "It defines the number of people you can have relationships of essentially trust and obligation with, as much as anything," Dunbar told the *Guardian* in 2010.[162] The Dunbar number of 150 can most easily be thought of as the number of people you *actively* keep in touch with. When I told Roger Neighbour about all this, he diligently applied that test to his entire Filofax and came back with a number of 148.

Although 150 is just an average, and particularly introverted or extroverted people will have social group sizes at the lower and higher extremes of the range, respectively, the implication of Dunbar's number being a limit is that when we exit one stage or phase of our lives and begin the next one, there is significant movement into and out of our group of meaningful contacts, which can feel difficult to cope with. University of Pennsylvania Professor of Philosophy Jennifer Morton writes in her book *Moving Up Without Losing Your Way*,

> When we lose people, communities and relationships that matter to us, they are not easily replaced. . . . Even if you then go on to make another friend as a result . . . the void left in your life by the first friend's passing isn't simply erased by the gain of the second friend. The resulting pain might be mitigated by the joys of making a new friend, but what you valued was that particular person in your life, and she can't simply be replaced by a new person.[163]

The best description I have found of this awareness of losing valued friends and the associated guilt is contained within *The Madness of Grief*, by the Reverend Richard Coles. He puts it better than I ever could when he writes,

> I had always felt bad about this, life choices of necessity relegating former priorities, and I missed them, not only because I loved them, but because as you live on you realise we are not so much the authors of our lives but a library of other people.[164]

Clearly no amount of anthropological understanding can remove the difficulty associated with the frequent making and losing of friendships, nor change the paradox that the more we enjoy our work and bond with our teams the harder the inevitable losses are to shoulder. But I do think that knowing we are confined by evolutionarily ancient neurobiological limits on our processing of social relationships can help us to go easy on ourselves, to feel less guilty for not getting round to making that call or sending that message, and equally to know that just because we have not heard from former colleagues and friends with whom we were once clinging to the same raft, it does not mean we have fallen in their estimations, are any less treasured or are any less loved. It is only that the loss is the price of goodbye.

In this final section, I have suggested that frequently changing jobs as part of a programme that we often have little or no control over can impose a significant psychological burden via the loss or high turnover of truly meaningful and valued relationships. It is one thing to contend with changes in our working lives that we have not necessarily chosen, but quite another to reach the stage of becoming responsible for our future professional directions, and by extension learning to live within a future we have chosen. The opportunity and indeed the necessity to start making career choices arrives quickly for new doctors, so in Chapter 7 we will discuss some different strategies for thinking about the impending medical crossroads.

"Tell me, what is it you plan to do
With your one wild and precious life?"

Mary Oliver, 'The Summer Day', from *House of Light*

7

SLIDING HOSPITAL DOORS

EARLY CAREER PLANNING AND MEDICAL WAYFINDING

Medical Crossroads

After just over a year of working post-qualification, UK doctors rapidly approach a decision point where they must decide whether to apply for specialty-training programmes, trust grade jobs, locum appointments, hospitals abroad or nothing medical at all. Time passes extremely quickly during the first year working as a doctor, and before you know it the point of choosing is on the horizon. Up until then, almost from the day you are accepted into medical school, you can ride along the medical conveyor belt, completing first university and then the UK Foundation Programme (or the international equivalents), until reaching the point that crystallises the fact that there is no career called 'Doctor'.

We vary widely in our reaction to these oncoming medical crossroads. Some young doctors have been set on a particular specialty for several years, feeling as sure that they want to be a hand surgeon, a GP, an obstetrician, a psychiatrist or a whichever other kind of doctor as they were that they wanted to study medicine in the first place. I count myself among them and in many senses, we are the lucky ones. A powerful sense of vocation with a desired and meaningful future goal can be a strong anchor when storms roll in, and a guiding compass when calmer seas allow us to move forwards. I tried to keep an open mind during medical school (and briefly thought about being a paediatrician), but really, I knew I wanted to work in anaesthetics and intensive care almost from the start. But for those who are unsure which medical specialty to pursue, the array of choices and the pressure to choose can be difficult.

I spoke to Georgia, a good friend from medical school, about how she was finding the process of career planning. "I really just don't know what I want to do," she told me.

> We get a little bit of time to do taster weeks in different specialties, but if you haven't actually done a full rotation in a specialty you might consider long-term, it can be quite tricky. Part of me thinks, is there something I haven't even thought about that I might enjoy?

Georgia is one of the most intelligent and kind junior doctors I know, and she manages to be both these things whilst simultaneously bringing up two young children. She is living evidence that brilliance is no guarantee of certainty in direction. The GMC currently recognises 65 specialties and 31 sub-specialties,[165] something that creates both exciting opportunities and a sometimes wicked choosing problem. Although lots of programmes keep options open (such as 'Internal Medicine Training' or 'Core Surgical Training' in the UK), it is easy to see how the plethora of choices gives rise to the fear of taking a wrong turn. We can worry that if we begin to train in the wrong specialty, we could feel out of place and all at sea.

This matters so much because square pegs in round holes do not for happy doctors make, and we have already seen in the previous chapter that our wellbeing is not to be taken for granted. What's more, the structure and requirements of modern training programmes mean that our career decisions, once made, are, although not irrevocable, extremely expensive in terms of time and money to reverse. It feels like finding the path that is right for us could hardly be more important. As I began to search for a way of thinking about the decisions that will shape our medical careers and our lives, I came across an intriguing concept. It is called Life Design.

Designing Your (Medical) Life

Bill Burnett and Dave Evans are the founders of the 'Life Design' course at Stanford University, in which they draw on their shared background in mechanical engineering and product design to apply design thinking principles to the question of how we can lead satisfying and meaningful lives. It has gone on to become one of the most popular courses at Stanford and was scientifically proven to work when two of the course's former students evaluated it for their PhD research.[166,167] In their book *Designing Your Life*, Burnett and Evans walk us through the techniques and mindsets taught on the Life Design course,[168] many of which could be useful when thinking about medical careers. The five core design tools they discuss are summarised in Table 7.1.

A further key concept elaborated by Burnett and Evans is that of the 'gravity problem'. "In life design", they write, "if it's not actionable then it's not a problem. It's a situation, a circumstance, a fact of life"[169]. They do make a theoretical distinction between problems that are totally inactionable (e.g. the existence of gravity) and problems that are 'functionally inactionable', meaning those that cannot realistically

Table 7.1 Applying Design Mindsets to Medical Career Planning

Design tool	*What is it?*	*Application*
Curiosity	A curious mindset helps us to see learning and opportunities in unexpected places. Staying curious helps people to "make their own luck".	Teaching, guidance and opportunities can arise when we least expect them. Career-enhancing and -enabling insights arrive when we stay curious.
Bias to Action	Trying stuff and being prepared to fail, rather than just thinking about the options. In product design, this is creating prototypes . . . and then more prototypes . . . and then some more.	How can we try out different specialties? This could be taster weeks, training rotations or out-of-programme jobs in specialties we're interested in.
Reframing	Taking new information about a problem, re-stating your position and starting over with new prototypes. Reframing helps us break away from dysfunctional beliefs, which are "myths that prevent people from designing the life they want".	Dysfunctional belief: "I have to find the specialty that's right for me." Reframe: "I need to try a variety of possible specialties that could be right for me."
Process Awareness	Awareness that we will all have ups and downs, triumphs and disasters, and that this is expected, in all of medicine as well as life. Nobody has it all worked out, and the journey is the destination.[170]	We can shorten our timelines to focus on the process of the days and weeks at hand, as we build forwards. With focus on the process, the long-term outcomes begin to take care of themselves.

Design tool	*What is it?*	*Application*
Radical Collaboration	Asking for help, a lot . . . and getting comfortable with doing so. Medicine is a team game. Seeking help widely is not a weakness, but a great strength.	Networking needn't be a dirty word. . . . Ask both near-peers and more senior colleagues to share their insights and experiences. Enlist collaborators. Build your team.

be addressed with the limits of the available time and resources, but overall the pair encourage people to avoid getting stuck fighting against an issue when there is nothing they can practically do about it. Burnett and Evans are careful not to come across as discouraging people from tackling very difficult but worthwhile problems, but emphasise that careful judgement is required before starting on a problem that will require a high input of time and effort with no guarantee of success.

When we approach medical crossroads gravity problems appear left and right, front and centre, and they usually have to do with application systems, how applicants are assessed and how training positions are allocated. "Why does the system have to make planning my life so difficult?" we all seem to be asking. Although these problems are theoretically actionable through structured consultations with the training administrators, trainee feedback and campaigns from medical unions (all of which are to be applauded), unless you are a medical student reading this chapter many years in advance of your own specialty decision point, they are functionally inactionable within the timeframe at hand. They are gravity problems.

One gravity problem in the UK is the geographical sizes of the areas trainees rotate within. In *This Is Going to Hurt*, the ex-obstetrics and gynaecology registrar turned comedian Adam Kay wrote,

> one such deanery is Kent, Surrey and Sussex: which I (and indeed the Ordnance Survey) had always considered to be three enormous, separate areas. Another deanery is Scotland. You know Scotland, that – what would you call it, oh yes – entire *country* measuring over 30,000 square miles.[171]

Another gravity problem is that beyond the UK Foundation Programme where coupled-up UK medical graduates can "link" their job applications, there is no mechanism for pairs of doctors in long-term relationships to have any guarantee of working anywhere near each other. These kinds of problems can be immensely frustrating, but accepting that they are gravity problems in the medical life design process is the only way to move forwards. Accepting that these problems are not actionable at present allows us to reframe the issue into something that is actionable. Some examples are shown in Box 7.1.

BOX 7.1 REFRAMING GRAVITY PROBLEMS IN MEDICAL LIFE DESIGN

GRAVITY PROBLEM: "Many of these deaneries are enormous and I would have no guarantee of where I would be working."

REFRAME: "Which deaneries can I apply to that have the highest proportion of locations within them that I would find acceptable?"

GRAVITY PROBLEM: "My girlfriend and I both want to do competitive specialties and we might not get training jobs in the same deanery."

REFRAME: "Which deaneries can we both apply to that include jobs located on the border with other deaneries (which we can simultaneously apply to)?"

Finding Balance

One of the most important reframes we need, I believe, is around the idea of work–life balance. When people speak about improving their work–life balance, most often what they are really talking about is trying to spend less time doing work and more time doing things they enjoy, with the people they love. The suggestion is that work and life are two separate and unrelated activities, and we would be happier if we could just find a way to do less of the former and more of the latter. It designates work as something negative that will not be enjoyable and will need to be counterbalanced by other things that can actually be counted as living. But work is an important part of our lives, and the term work–life balance is unhelpful in the way that it puts a downer on work from the get-go, casting it into a hinterland outside of enjoyable life, as something to be endured only out of necessity.

Work, and medicine in particular, can be physically and emotionally exhausting, and of course we all need time to rest, to relax and to recharge our batteries. But even if we switch to using the more accurate term 'work–leisure balance', I am still not sure that numerically assessing which options afford the most leisure time is the best way to evaluate potential careers. We can do better than this. We can be more optimistic and more hopeful for the role of work in our lives than thinking from the negative perspective of how it can best be "balanced out". We should search for work that is nourishing and enriching, work that helps us to grow rather than depleting us. "I am looking for a specialty with great work–life balance" can be reframed as "I am looking for a specialty I'll love working in that fits well with the rest of my life."

The late Paul Kalanithi wrote in *When Breath Becomes Air*, "Putting lifestyle first is how you find a job – not a calling"[172]. At first glance, it seems that Kalanithi was simply arguing that a true vocation for a medical specialty should trump lifestyle (a.k.a. 'leisure time') considerations when it comes to career decisions, perhaps to justify his thousands of hours spent training to become a neurosurgeon. Yet an alternative reading of his words is that achieving a sense of vocation with work that is truly meaningful to us is a more reliable route to happiness than any strategy built around the idea of work–life balance. If we find a career path that we have deeply connected with, where our work and the other parts of our life that matter can be mutually supporting and reinforcing, the need to counterbalance our work melts away. So how can we find these elusive paths?

Wayfinding

In *Designing Your Life*, Burnett and Evans introduce the concept of "wayfinding", which they define as "the ancient art of figuring out where you are going when you don't actually know your destination"[173]. If you're thinking that this all sounds a bit fantastical and wondering how on earth this could help with medical career decisions, hang on in there for now! The authors go on to explain that rather than a detailed map with a known destination (which can't exist for our future careers and lives), what we actually need and *can* have is a "compass" to get us heading in the right direction. They suggest that we can reflect on the different types of work we're doing and rate the work based on our levels of engagement and energy, using an AEIOU mnemonic to structure the reflection thinking about Activities, Environments, Interactions, Objects and Users (designer speak for the people involved in the work).

Using this kind of reflective process could be a good way to work out what it is that we like or don't like about medical work that we *have* done, and then use that to inform our subsequent steps for what to try next that we *haven't* done. It can guide us to continue with what we're doing or to change tack. It can set our direction. One SHO I spoke to realised that she really enjoyed doing practical procedures but didn't like operating theatres and also didn't want to give up the diagnostic challenge of being a physician. She therefore started working towards specialising in gastroenterology, where she could become both a skilled endoscopist and diagnostician. I mentioned earlier that I considered a career in paediatrics for a while, but I eventually realised that I was not any more interested in children's medicine than adult medicine, and didn't particularly enjoy clinic work either. What I had been engaged and energised by was the care of acutely sick children, who can deteriorate rapidly when their physiological compensation reaches its limits. This reflection set me back onto Plan A, which was critical care.

If we have begun to get an idea of our direction, even without having a map or knowing the final destination, we can brainstorm prototypes to explore by doing an exercise Burnett and Evans call "Odyssey planning". Odyssey plans, they propose, are distinctly different possible versions of the next five years of our lives. "One of the most powerful ways to design your life is to design your lives," they argue.[174] The Odyssey plans each need to be reasonably different to get the most value from this exercise, so sketching out three possible lives as an oesophageal surgeon, a hepatobiliary surgeon and a colorectal surgeon is probably cheating! A worksheet to help with the process is freely available on www.designingyour.life in the resources section.[175]

The idea of Odyssey planning reminded me of a novel I read aged 18, on the verge of leaving home to start medical school. In Herman Hesse's *The Glass Bead Game* (translated from the original German title *Das Glasperlenspiel*), we follow the life of a young scholar named Joseph Knecht living in the 23rd century Kingdom of Castalia. There, the scholars attempt to master "The Glass Bead Game", a feat requiring the integration and fusion of multiple diverse areas of human knowledge. One of the exercises they are set during their apprenticeship is to write three "lives" for themselves, these "lives" each being stories imagining how their life might have played out had they been born in an entirely different era, place or culture. As I set out on the path I had chosen, Hesse's novel was the first nudge I encountered towards the understanding that we could each lead several different lives.[176]

Our Endless Possible Lives

In the same way that there isn't actually 'the one' love of our life, and there are in fact many (albeit hard to find) people we may love, the truth when it comes to the big choices is that amongst our endless possible lives there will be a great number that are right. The idea that there is one best option to be reached, if only we could determine what it is and then find the way to get there, can lead to a kind of decision paralysis where we are afraid to commit wholly to one path for fear of missing out on something better. Applied in retrospect, this same way of thinking can cause profound regret and unhappiness if we are saddled with thoughts of, "If only I'd done x rather than y" or "If only I'd chosen a over b", then wouldn't everything have turned out differently?

Of course, things would have been different, but they may not have been better. In Matt Haig's novel *The Midnight Library*, a young woman named Nora Seed tries to take her own life after losing her job compounds her depression, but she wakes up neither dead nor alive in a dream-like place called 'The Midnight Library'[177]. The library contains row upon row of books, stretching farther than the eye can see, with each one containing a different life that Nora could have led had she chosen differently at some stage. What if she'd stuck with her swimming training? What if her band had secured a record contract? What if she'd gone with her friend to Australia? The librarian, who incidentally takes the form of Nora's childhood school librarian, Mrs Elm, tells her that she can open any of these books, experience and live in that version of her life, and ultimately stay living within that alternative version if it is what she truly desires. But if at any point she realises that she does not in fact want that alternative life, she will immediately find herself back in the Midnight Library.

Haig invokes multiverse theory and the idea of parallel lives within infinite parallel worlds as a prism through which to challenge the dysfunctional belief that there is one perfect life for each of us, which we may have missed out on. As Nora explores and lives through many of her possible lives, it becomes clear that they all have their fair share of happiness and sadness, of joy and despair. When she is asked by an interviewer in her life as a famous (but troubled) rock star if she ever wonders what her life would have been like if she had decided to take a different path, she replies,

> I think it's easy to imagine there are easier paths . . . but maybe there are no easy paths. . . . We spend so much time wishing our lives were different, comparing ourselves to other people and to other versions of ourselves, when really most lives contain degrees of good and degrees of bad.[178]

By the end of the novel, when Nora has returned to her original life in Bedford and is recovering from her overdose, she writes,

> It is easy to mourn the lives we aren't living. Easy to wish we had developed other talents, said yes to different offers. . . . It is not difficult to see yourself through the lens of other people, and to wish you were all the different kaleidoscopic versions of you they wanted you to be. . . . But it is not our lives we regret not living that are the real problem. It is the regret itself.[179]

Haig concludes in the penultimate chapter, "The prison wasn't the place but the perspective"[180].

The lessons from *The Midnight Library* are universal, but are particularly relevant for mapping medical careers where we are faced with both a vast array of possibilities and significant uncertainty regarding our chances of actually securing our preferred options. The majority of the public do not appreciate the fact that young doctors cannot simply choose a specialty and a location and then get on with it. Especially for doctors interested in competitive specialties who have partners, children or other dependents, it sometimes becomes necessary to compromise on one or both of specialty choice and location. Of course, we should try to build the career that is right for us, sample widely if necessary and find work that will be meaningful and enjoyable not only in the long term, but also in the process of getting there. Our current lives matter greatly, more if anything than our future possible lives, and the journey is the destination. But in choosing our next steps we should be reassured and comforted that perfect does not exist. There is no perfect location. Certainly, there is no easy specialty. All of medicine, and indeed life, brings its triumphs and disasters, its elation and despair, and more of it is random than we would like to believe. Yes, we can plan and design our lives, but our power as architects has its limits. Realising and accepting this, I have found, can make us much happier as we journey onwards.

But what if, life design exercises complete and all things considered, you reach the conclusion that a possible life away from clinical medicine, or perhaps away from medicine altogether, holds the most appeal? There will be no shortage of senior doctors, friends or family lining up to gently (or not so gently) suggest reconsidering, or to take more time, or to give just one more specialty a try. They are right to urge both caution and consideration of how trying alternative careers will impact upon things like professional registration and revalidation, yet for a small but significant number of young doctors leaving medicine may truly be a good path. There could be many upsides of quitting.

The Upsides of Quitting

It may seem surprising, perverse even, in a book concerned with patient safety to include a section discussing the option for young doctors to leave medicine altogether. Why mention this choice when NHS hospitals are already beleaguered by chronic understaffing and rota gaps, with the UK having one of the lowest doctors per capita ratios in Europe?[181] Plainly there are few things as important to patient safety as having an adequate number of doctors to look after the patients. Why not focus on persuading them all to stay? The truth is that almost all of us, even if only on the worst of days, will have had the upsides of quitting cross our minds. And whilst leaving is only a passing thought for the majority of doctors, for some it grows into a serious possibility that demands to be considered. In a discussion of wayfinding through our careers, it would be doing a gross disservice to those colleagues to push the option under the carpet. Medicine is not a cult with a one-way entry system. We all have the right to walk away.

The title of this section is borrowed from an episode of the *Freakonomics Radio* podcast, which discusses the yin and yang of sunk costs and opportunity costs when thinking about quitting.[182] In this context, sunk costs can be thought of as any irretrievable time, effort or financial resources that have been put into reaching a particular point on a career path. In medical careers, the sunk costs are extreme. For example, at the time of writing I have spent eight years and ten months as either a medical student or post-graduate doctor, have studied for and passed 43 examinations and still have a student debt balance of £72,698. When these sunk costs are put forward as an argument against quitting, i.e. sticking with the status quo, it is referred to in behavioural economics as the 'Sunk Costs Fallacy'. These costs are long gone and we can't get them back, so someone entirely unbiased by sunk costs would regard them as irrelevant to the choice at hand. In reality, it doesn't feel that easy.

Opportunity costs, on the other hand, are the costs to us of *not* quitting, of *not* changing paths and therefore missing out on the opportunities of an alternative. We can't properly weigh up the value of a choice in isolation from the next best option, because we incur a cost from the missed benefits of the option we reject. Opportunity costs are essentially behavioural economics speak for measuring our FOMO. The part about comparing a preferred choice to the 'next best option' is really important; it would be an easy mistake to subconsciously factor in the opportunity costs of *all* the myriad options you don't select, but you could never have gone for all of them anyway. If we incorrectly count the opportunity costs of multiple possible alternatives, we will either be very unhappy with our choice or never choose at all. We could be paralysed in our status quo. Furthermore, in *The Paradox of Choice*, Barry Schwartz reminds us, "The existence of multiple alternatives makes it easy for us to imagine alternatives that don't exist – alternatives that combine the attractive features of the ones that do exist"[183]. It is true that if we are mentally building Eden from components of many different gardens, then the grass will always be greener.

I spoke to a friend called Tom, a doctor who has put a great deal of thought into whether he should leave medicine in order to try an alternative career. "In my first year I had mainly surgical rotations, which I didn't enjoy at all and I knew I didn't want to be a surgeon," Tom told me.

> And by my haematology rotation, which was my second job in second year, I was having thoughts about quitting medicine. I had started to become more aware of the systemic problems relating to how the system treats junior doctors, outside of department-specific or specialty-specific things.

He went on to eloquently explain the concept of an "exploit versus explore" choice dilemma, which relates to the age-old question of whether to stick or twist. Tom posited,

> If you want to get a takeaway tonight, do you go for a tried-and-tested favourite or try something new? There are values to both, but it's also true that for an individual the total amount of time you can enjoy something is limited. As you get older, the value of exploring new things drops and the value of exploiting something you already have or already know about increases. If you're in your twenties, the value of exploring something is much higher.

Put differently, if you've been seriously considering quitting medicine, the opportunity costs of staying put could be significant.

However, one thing that Tom was also very clear on was that it's important for people considering quitting to be clear in their own minds about the causative factors behind their current emotional state. It can be easy to misattribute negative feelings to the demands of working in medicine if other factors are at play.

> If you're thinking about a career change because you're unhappy, but you're also going through a really difficult break-up, that's probably a good time to just take a step back, to breathe, and to be careful about how you're assigning causes to things. For me, I had so many reasons to be unhappy outside of my career. I was in a long-distance relationship with my girlfriend who I wasn't getting to see because of the Covid lockdown, I couldn't do my hobbies, I was stuck in the flat and the whole weeks were go to work, come home, eat, sleep and repeat. And any job, in that context, was going to be a bit unpleasant.

So, Tom tried to optimise everything he could. He got scientific about it, made some changes, ready to look again to see if he felt any better. "For this reason, I feel good about deciding to have another year as a doctor, to see if I can improve things," he explained.

> I'm moving in with my girlfriend, moving back down south to be closer to university friends, lockdown is lifting meaning I can socialise more and pursue hobbies, I'll try another specialty I may enjoy and the commute will be shorter. If after optimising all of that I'm still having thoughts about leaving medicine, then that's a good experiment that I've run.

The Incredibly Difficult Problem

So before deciding on leaving for definite, it seems sensible to first do everything you can to see if staying could be better. But there remains what Tom calls "The Incredibly Difficult Problem" for those weighing up whether or not to continue in medicine. We are consistently told that things will be better once training is over and we have become consultants, meaning that to these ends we should tolerate the years of gruelling rotations around widely spread hospitals, desperately struggling to keep the other relationships and parts of our lives afloat as we go. These intensely challenging years will all be worth it to be a consultant since "you'll be a consultant for more than three times as long as you're a trainee", the argument goes.

This way of thinking is flawed, however, because it assumes that potential future time is of equal value to the present time available to us *right now*. It is not. It cannot be. Even without the somewhat morbid (but totally valid) perspective that any of us could die tomorrow in a tragic accident, the higher value of present time compared with future time can be easily demonstrated. Assuming that you're a young doctor in your twenties, would you be prepared to pay £5000 now in order to receive £1 million on the day you turn 50? Provided that you have some savings to invest into this deal, most people will answer yes. Would you be prepared to pay £5000 now to receive £1 million on the day you turn 60? There will probably be some disagreement on this one, but personally I'd still take the offer. Would you be prepared to pay £5000 now in order to receive £1 million on the day you turn 85? Absolutely not. Why? Because being both alive and well enough to enjoy the money by that age is so far from guaranteed that it's not worth your £5000 investment. The greater our degree of certainty both of reaching a given period of time and regarding our life situation when we get there, the more valuable that time should be to us. There really is no time like the present.

If present time is so much more valuable than future time, why knuckle down and work for anything? Why don't we just pack it all in and live for the moment? Did the seasonaires who spent their summers on the beach in Vasiliki and their winters on the slopes of Val d'Isère whilst we were passing exam after exam at medical school have it right all along? They may have done. But crucially, that depends on whether working hard and playing hard doing seasons was what they truly wanted to be doing, just as much as it depends on whether studying and then training in medicine was what we truly wanted to be doing. Having understood that present time is more valuable than future time, the logical next step (rather than heading out on an all-night bender) is to re-assess, and perhaps search for, the meaning to be found in our everyday work, the things that anchor us to why we are there even when the challenges become tumultuous. It is not sensible, or sustainable, to continue on a path only because "next year" or "when you're a consultant" things might be better. Whilst the higher value of present time might frame exactly why some doctors feel they cannot continue in medicine, it is equally an angle that can refocus us on the things that we do love about being doctors. The Incredibly Difficult Problem of feeling as though we're trading off current happiness for potential future happiness can only be solved by re-finding purpose and meaning in the journey, however long and difficult the path.

Walking Away

Many doctors do eventually decide to leave clinical practice. The *Student BMJ* podcast 'Sharp Scratch' interviewed Fiona Godlee, editor of the BMJ, about her decision to switch from working as a doctor to being an editor.[184] She discussed the way in which our professional and personal identities are often intertwined, and how the period of separation can be prolonged.

> Changing your identity internally was tricky . . . for a long time I said to people, 'I'm a doctor, but I'm currently working as an editor.' It took me about five years to stop saying that, because a doctor is something so substantial and so concrete. Then I began to say, 'I used to be a doctor and now I'm an editor' and then I stopped even bothering to say that.

Fiona Godlee also highlighted the fact that it is not easy to leave a role with a high social status, one which some doctors may have initially leant towards due to pressure from family or other reasons beyond a personal sense of vocation for medicine. "It can take a lot of courage to move away from a role that you've taken on for the wrong reasons," she affirmed, adding, "I would applaud people who do that."

I agree that the courage to quit is something to be celebrated. There will be critics who argue that the state subsidising a medical degree means this shouldn't be the case, that these doctors knew what they were signing up for and should see their training through. But did any of us really know, in a meaningful sense, what becoming a doctor would be like? I was thorough. I did my research. I read Max Pemberton and Atul Gawande and everything I could get my hands on. Yet it does not prepare you for the reality of the work – the holding fast with a patient after a chilling diagnosis, the sensation of ribs cracking beneath your hands at a cardiac arrest or the knowledge that the pen you prescribe with could be a lethal weapon. Even if some doctors did start out for the wrong reasons, it is equally likely that for others the reasons which felt right at the time just don't feel right anymore. It cannot be the case that 100% of the people who thought aged 17 that they wanted to be a doctor were correct. Millions of years of evolution have given us a human brain that, when asked how much we will change in the future, tends to underestimate. It is unfair to blame young doctors for that.

I began this discussion of quitting medicine defending its right to be included. I hope that it has been valuable for some readers, perhaps not only for those thinking of leaving altogether, but for anyone weighing up whether to leave their current specialty and begin the long journey of retraining in a different one. I mentioned the importance of workforce retention for patient safety, but I would equally pose the safety-focused question of "Would you want your loved ones, or yourself, to be treated by a doctor who no longer wants to be there?" What's more, it is my hope that even if some readers of this section do go on to leave medicine, at least as many who were wavering may choose to pause, to reconsider and eventually to stay with us. Both groups should have our respect.

For those who are leaving medicine, or changing specialty or undergoing an upheaval in any other aspect of life, I think the conclusion from an episode of the *Hidden Brain* podcast titled "Loss and Renewal" has much to offer.[185] Host Shankar Vedantam reflected:

> All of us have chapters in our lives that close, and when they do, especially if it's a chapter we have known and loved for a long time, it can feel like the whole book is over, that there's nothing left to do, maybe even nothing left to live for. But I think each of us has stories in our lives that reflect the fact that the people we are today are not the same people we were a few years ago. We often underestimate our capacity to re-invent ourselves.

I have listened to these words time and again. We can take great comfort in our chances for renewal.

CONCLUSION

IT'S ABOUT TIME

More than four years have passed since my Black Wednesday, and it has been more than two and a half years since I sat down in mid-December 2019 and planned what has become *The Bleep Test*. A few weeks after tapping out that Word document, with no idea if I would ever get round to doing anything with it, the world began to change quite dramatically and before long writing a book couldn't have been further from my mind. Yet as the routines of pandemic working settled into place, in both the first and second waves of Covid-19 I often found myself with unfilled hours alone in the flat and time to think about our work, the position new doctors are put in and the transformation we undergo. It seemed that time was on my side. I had time to read more than I had in years. I became interested in cognitive and social psychology, behavioural economics, evolutionary biology and anthropology – the human sciences – and realised that they have quite a lot to say about the difficulties new doctors encounter, and sometimes some solutions to offer. Doctors are humans too, after all.

But time was marching on, and with every month that passed since my Black Wednesday, I was getting further away from walking in the shoes of the people who *The Bleep Test* is primarily intended to help. Sure, I could remember events and anecdotes from those early months, but it was getting harder to recall the *feeling* of what it is like to be so completely new to the responsibility of doctoring and to be so inexperienced. For this reason, I have tried not to edit or rewrite much of the first half of the book, which was written when I was somewhat closer to day zero than I am now. This passing of time seemed as good a reason as any to hurry up and try to finish writing, but it speaks to a central point about how we care for new doctors and understand what is needed to keep both them and our patients safe. In the same way that SHOs sometimes struggle to verbalise for a medical student each of the steps required to insert a cannula, or anaesthetists have to pause and think to explain their seamless intubation of the trachea, we all forget how much we have learned. We forget how far we have come.

A couple of weeks after the August changeover, my friend Mike and his fiancée were round for dinner. Mike was telling my flatmate and me how difficult he was finding it to supervise the new doctors on his ward. "I know they're still very new," he said, "But I do sort of despair – today, for example, I found that none of the Chronic Liver Disease (CLD) patients in Bay 3 have had Enoxaparin for VTE prophylaxis for four days!" This decision, to prescribe or not prescribe a prophylactic blood thinner in liver patients, requires the specific hepatology knowledge that impaired liver production of physiological *anti-coagulants* such as Protein C (as well as impaired production of clotting factors) means that, in general, they are actually in a relatively pro-thrombotic state. Unless the patient is actively bleeding, the Enoxaparin is usually indicated. Clots kill you faster than bleeds. "The thing is Mike, I definitely didn't know that in my first year post-qualification," I mused. "It's a blind spot for them, I'm sure they thought they were doing the right thing."

In Chapter 1, we saw how the Dunning–Kruger blind spot bias of not knowing what we don't know is one of the trickiest problems when it comes to how new doctors can get things right. Here, we have come across a related, but arguably even more important, problem of senior doctors not knowing what new doctors don't know. Assumptions rarely end well. Where do we go from here? How should we make things better for new doctors? The answer definitely is not, as Mike's senior registrar disturbingly told him, "to sometimes let things go to shit so that they learn faster". Would he say that if it was his own mother on the ward? Secondly, the answer also isn't to review the undergraduate hepatology curriculum, ensure that VTE risk assessment in CLD patients is included and add a question in the MCQ paper at finals for good measure. Education is important, but medicine is so vast that we will all, always, have blind spots throughout our careers. We cannot educate our way to zero harm, the patient safety goal Jeremy Hunt advocates in *Zero: Eliminating Unnecessary Deaths in a Post-pandemic NHS* not because absolute zero is truly possible but because "if we reject this as an ambition, our actions are destined to fall short of the potential for change"[186].

What about emphasising the risks of cognitive biases to new doctors? Shouldn't we get them all to think about how they may not know what they don't know? Whilst it is true that you will never take steps to mitigate the risks of a cognitive bias you've never heard of, and Groopman's assertion we heard in Chapter 1 that doctors should "be schooled in heuristics – in the power and necessity of shortcuts, and in their pitfalls and dangers"[187] is correct, just thinking a lot about thinking won't cut the mustard. When Daniel Kahneman was asked about having studied cognitive biases for more than half a century, he remarked,

> I'm considered one of the worst offenders on many of these mistakes. . . . Some people read *Thinking, Fast and Slow* in the hope that reading it will improve their minds. I wrote it, and it didn't improve my mind. Those things (cognitive biases) are deep and they're powerful and they're hard to change.[188]

No, what we really have to do is build systems across our institutions that acknowledge and account for the fact that new doctors are new, their teams and supervisors are imperfect and that humans will always be, well, human. We need to include multiple layers of failsafes. Mike's ward actually had an electronic prescribing system available, but the processes in place were not sensible, with doctors still having the option to prescribe on paper if they hadn't admitted the patient electronically. Two different systems in play on the same ward sounded like a recipe for drug errors. "Ok, so why not start by agreeing with everyone in the department that only the electronic prescribing system will be used when patients land on the ward?" I suggested. The next thing would be to work with the consultants to update and improve the electronic decision support for VTE prophylaxis in liver patients. After that, you could add a ward round checklist to nudge teams to review the drug charts. Systems, not individuals, make for safer patients.

If the system is the key, what about the macro-level systemic factors that affect everything all doctors, not just new ones, are able to do to help patients? We saw in Chapter 4, for example, the deficiencies in rest facilities for staff doing difficult shift work, and in Chapters 5 and 6, considered how much more needs to be done to protect the psychological wellbeing of those doing caring work. Yet more generally, at the time of writing, it is fair to say that the UK healthcare system is in a dire state. Patient satisfaction is falling, elective surgical waiting times are substantial, and the ambulance service is on its knees, overwhelmed with desperate calls for help. Corridor medicine has become the norm in Emergency Departments nationwide. Patients wait unconscionably long durations for the privilege of being examined in makeshift cubicles behind plastic screens. Privacy and dignity have become luxury items. And the ambulances queue outside, sometimes with deteriorating patients kept aboard when there's no room at the inn. Working conditions have never been more challenging, and amongst all this chaos new doctors are in danger of being overlooked and overwhelmed.

The Bleep Test is not intended to be a political book, so I have tried not to labour these points in the preceding chapters. It would not be difficult to roll out pages of prose detailing the extent of the crisis, with numerous statistics and references to back it all up. The prevailing conditions, however, are so blindingly obvious that I don't think it is unreasonable to accept these as a given. They are the setting of this story. Of course, it matters immensely that doctors continue to campaign loudly and persistently on these issues, highlighting that problems such as underfunding and understaffing are chief amongst all patient safety concerns. But that is not what *The Bleep Test* is about. I have tried to follow the philosophy of Dan Dworkis' *The Emergency Mind* that we should "rapidly accept reality" in order to usefully move forwards and make our next moves.[189] For the new doctor starting out, these system-wide problems are, for the moment, gravity problems. You will remember from Chapter 7 that "gravity problems" are those which are not solvable with the time and resources currently available. The question at hand is how we negotiate this incredibly challenging environment in a positive and hopeful way. Whilst many of the psychological problems we have discussed are intrinsic to the learning curve of medicine and would be there even in the best of systems, it is a question of degrees. It is even harder to keep your head when all around you seem to be losing theirs. I hope that some of the tools and ways of thinking in this book might be helpful, but equally hope that, one day, *The Bleep Test* will feel much less necessary than it does right now. It will be about time, too.

There are a few risks in writing a book like this one. The first is misrepresenting the issues *The Bleep Test* contends with as simply being one final section of knowledge – the hidden curriculum – that is easily mastered, if only it can be unveiled. It may seem as though I naively believe I have collected enough experience to have all the answers – that I work blissfully content, thinking I have mastered the hidden curriculum and should therefore be the one to make it un-hidden. The truth, of course, is that I have collected enough experience only to start asking the right questions. At times I have been over-confident when I was wrong, and at other times have been under-confident when I was right. In *Letters to a Young Poet*, the Austrian novelist and poet Rainer Maria Rilke urges his young correspondent:

> Do not believe that he who seeks to comfort you lives untroubled amongst the simple and quiet words that sometimes do you good. His life has much difficulty and sadness and remains far behind yours. Were it otherwise, he would never have been able to find those words.[190]

So, it is the same with *The Bleep Test*. I haven't got it all figured out, and I live still troubled amongst these issues. I am still learning, still struggling, still stumbling. I have found these words only because I do not have all the answers.

The process of switching from medical student to new doctor can be imagined and prepared for in advance but can only be realised by living through those days. There is no way around it, but we can alter the mindset with which we go through it. And perhaps we can also alter the mindset of those who will be alongside us, supporting us, holding space for us whilst, with time, we begin to emerge. And emerge we all will.

A few weeks before leaving the University Spaceship, I bumped into Marco, one of the Advanced Clinical Practitioners who had been there for me in my first job, back at the very start. "Luke!" he exclaimed. "How are you doing?" We chatted for a while, leaning against the wall as the daily comings and goings of the critical care corridor passed us by. Behind the wall the relentless work of the pandemic wore on, but for a brief moment we were away from it all, looking across the city through the glass, across the rooftops towards the District General Hospital, and across the time that had passed since we first met. "It's so good to see you now," Marco said. "All grown up, and happy and settled. I remember when you were a brand new doctor!" And so did I.

ACKNOWLEDGEMENTS

I owe a huge amount of thanks to all the friends and colleagues I have studied and worked with over the past ten years – too many to name but you know who you are. I'm humbled to call so many of you friends. To everyone who has supervised and trained me, I hope that this book will manage to pass on to others some of what you taught me.

Thank you to Tom Frost, Aybuke Atalay, Matt Tranter, Anne Berkeley, Joe Spearing, Gina Hadley, David Matthews, Ashok Handa, Daryl Menezes, Lois Brand, Mum, Dad and Jo, all of whom read various sections and provided thoughtful criticism and encouragement.

Ali Tomlin helped me hugely with the cover design, even when we changed the book's title at the eleventh hour and went back to the drawing board. Thank you to Jo for suggesting the excellent new title in less than two minutes, after I had spent more than two months thinking about the previous one.

Henry Marsh kindly allowed me to quote a response from a live question-and-answer session in Blackwell's Bookshop the best part of a decade ago. Scott Weingart similarly allowed me to reproduce his comments about medical error that had originally existed in podcast form. Matt Walton was generous in allowing me to retell his story in Chapter 5, and offered plenty of encouragement and food for thought.

Thank you to the team at CRC Press/Taylor & Francis including Jo Koster, Linda Leggio and Neha Bhatt, and to Spandana P B, Manoranjan and Nitya at Apex CoVantage, for all of your hard work making the book become a reality. Thank you also to Caroline Lalley, who did a thorough and meticulous copy edit of the manuscript.

Thank you to Parveen Kumar for writing such an excellent Foreword to the book. I am very grateful.

Finally, I am especially grateful to Roger Neighbour, who not only read each chapter and encouraged me to carry on with the next one, but has been a tireless source of friendship and support. Roger, I am sure *The Bleep Test* would not have happened without you.

ABBREVIATIONS

A&E	Accident and Emergency
ALS	Advanced Life Support
AMU	Acute Medical Unit
BMA	British Medical Association
BMJ	*British Medical Journal*
CCOT	Critical Care Outreach Team
CLD	Chronic Liver Disease
CPR	CardioPulmonary Resuscitation
CRM	Crew Resource Management
CT	Computed Tomography
DCT	Dual Cognition Theory
DGH	District General Hospital
DNACPR	Do Not Attempt CardioPulmonary Resuscitation
EM	Emergency Medicine
ED	Emergency Department
FOMO	Fear Of Missing Out
GCS	Glasgow Coma Scale

GHQ-12	General Health Questionnaire (twelve-item)
GMC	General Medical Council
GP	General Practitioner
HDU	High Dependency Unit
ICU	Intensive Care Unit
IM	Intramuscular
INR	International Normalised Ratio
IV	Intravenous
MCQ	Multiple Choice Question
NHS	National Health Service
NICU	Neonatal Intensive Care Unit
PEG	Percutaneous Endoscopic Gastrostomy
PEPS	Performance-Enhancing Psychological Skills
PPE	Personal Protective Equipment
PTSD	Post Traumatic Stress Disorder
PVT	Psychomotor Vigilance Test
RCT	Randomised Controlled Trial
SHO	Senior House Officer
TSMB	Targeted Stretching Micro-Break
VTE	Venous Thromboembolism
WHO	World Health Organisation

NOTES

Introduction – Black Wednesday

1 Jen MH, Bottle A, Majeed A, Bell D, Aylin P. Early in-hospital mortality following trainee doctors' first day at work. PLoS ONE. 2009; 4(9). doi:10.1371/journal.pone.0007103

2 Rimmer A. 60 seconds on . . . Black Wednesday. BMJ. 2017; j3574. doi:10.1136/bmj.j3574

3 Rifkin-Zybutz RP, Taylor T, Spencer JI. Re: 60 seconds on . . . Black Wednesday. British Medical Journal. 2017; 358:3574. doi:10.1136/bmj.j3574

4 Dillner L. Frightening realism. BMJ. 1994; 308(6936):1108. doi:10.1136/bmj.308.6936.1108

5 Aylin P, Majeed FA. The killing season – Fact or fiction? BMJ. 1994; 309(6970):1690. doi:10.1136/bmj.309.6970.1690

6 Jena B, Elliot D. Episode 44: Why is July a bad month to visit the hospital? [Internet]. 2022. Available from: https://freakonomics.com/podcast/why-is-july-a-bad-month-to-visit-the-hospital/

7 Young JQ, Ranji SR, Wachter RM, Lee CM, Niehaus B, Auerbach AD. "July effect": Impact of the academic year-end changeover on patient outcomes — A systematic review. Annals of Internal Medicine. 2011; 155(5):309–15. doi:10.7326/0003-4819-155-5-201109060-00354

8 Haller G, Myles PS, Taffe P, Perneger TV, Wu CL. Rate of undesirable events at beginning of academic year: Retrospective cohort study. BMJ. 2009; 339:b3974. doi:10.1136/bmj.b3974
9 Hope J. 'Killing season' on NHS wards: Patients at risk when junior doctors start new jobs, says health boss. Daily Mail [Internet]. 2012 June 22; Available from: https://www.dailymail.co.uk/news/article-2163382/NHS-wards-Patients-risk-junior-doctors-start-new-jobs-says-health-boss-Sir-Bruce-Keogh
10 Anderson DJ. The hidden curriculum. American Journal of Roentgenology. 1992; 159:21–2. doi:10.2214/ajr.159.1.1609700
11 Lempp H, Seale C. The hidden curriculum in undergraduate medical education: Qualitative study of medical students' perceptions of teaching. BMJ. 2004; 329(7469):770–3. doi:10.1136/bmj.329.7469.770

Chapter 1: Decisions, Decisions

12 NHS England. Patient safety [Internet]. NHS England website. Available from: https://www.england.nhs.uk/patient-safety/
13 Groopman J. How Doctors Think (First Mariner Books edition). Boston: Houghton Mifflin Company; 2008, p. 67.
14 Levitin D. The Organized Mind. London: Penguin Random House; 2015.
15 Levitin D. The Organized Mind. London: Penguin Random House; 2015, p. 16.
16 Levitin D. The Organized Mind. London: Penguin Random House; 2015, p. 35.
17 Clarke R. Your Life in My Hands (Kindle edition). Metro Publishing; 2017, pp. 104–20.
18 Kahneman D. Thinking, Fast and Slow. London: Penguin Books Ltd; 2012.
19 General Medical Council. Good Medical Practice. Manchester: General Medical Council; 2020.
20 Rowling J. K. Harry Potter and the Chamber of Secrets (Kindle edition). Pottermore Publishing; 2015, p. 279.
21 General Medical Council. Outcomes for Provisionally Registered Doctors with a License to Practise (The Trainee Doctor). Manchester: General Medical Council; 2015.

22 Kruger J, Dunning D. Unskilled and unaware of it: How difficulties in recognizing one's own incompetence lead to inflated self-assessments. Journal of Personality and Social Psychology. 1999; 77(6):1121–34. doi:10.1037/0022-3514.77.6.1121
23 Luft J, Ingham H. The Johari window, a graphic model of interpersonal awareness. Proceedings of the Western Training Laboratory in Group Development. Los Angeles: UCLA, 1955.
24 Syed M. Rebel Ideas: The Power of Diverse Thinking. London: John Murray; 2019.
25 Phillips KW, Northcraft GB, Neale MA. Surface-level diversity and decision-making in groups: When does deep-level similarity help? Group Processes & Intergroup Relations. 2006; 9(4):467–82. doi:10.1177/1368430206067557
26 Morgan M. Critical: Stories from the Front Line of Intensive Care Medicine. London: Simon & Schuster; 2019, pp. 74–5.
27 Giles L. The Art of War by Sun Tzu (Special Edition). London: Special Edition Books; 2007.
28 Adams E, Goyder C, Heneghan C, Brand L, Ajjawi R. Clinical reasoning of junior doctors in emergency medicine: A grounded theory study. Emergency Medicine Journal. 2017; 34(2):70–5. doi:10.1136/emermed-2015-205650
29 Croskerry P. Achieving quality in clinical decision making: Cognitive strategies and detection of bias. Academic Emergency Medicine. 2002; 9(11):1184–204. doi:10.1111/j.1553-2712.2002.tb01574.x
30 Morgenstern J. Cognitive errors in medicine: The common errors [Internet]. First10EM. 2015. Available from: https://first10em.com/cognitive-errors
31 Groopman J. How Doctors Think (First Mariner Books edition). Boston: Houghton Mifflin Company; 2008, p. 273.
32 Groopman J. How Doctors Think (First Mariner Books edition). Boston: Houghton Mifflin Company; 2008, p. 36.
33 Mamede S, Schmidt HG, Rikers RMJP, Penaforte JC, Coelho-Filho JM. Influence of perceived difficulty of cases on physicians' diagnostic reasoning. Academic Medicine. 2008; 83(12):1210–6. doi:10.1097/ACM.0b013e31818c71d7
34 Yerkes RM, Dodson JD. The relation of strength of stimulus to rapidity of habit-formation. Journal of Comparative Neurology and Psychology. 1908; 18(5):459–82. doi:10.1002/cne.920180503

35 Hearns S. Peak Performance under Pressure: Lessons from a Helicopter Rescue Doctor (Kindle edition). Bridgwater: Class Professional Publishing; 2019, p. 20.
36 Hearns S. Peak Performance under Pressure: Lessons from a Helicopter Rescue Doctor (Kindle edition). Bridgwater: Class Professional Publishing; 2019, p. 15.
37 Osler W. Aequanimitas. London: Ravenio Books; 1927.

Chapter 2: Accidental Emergencies

38 Syed M. Black Box Thinking: Marginal Gains and the Secret of High Performance. London: John Murray; 2015, p. 35
39 Marsh H. Do No Harm: Stories of Life, Death and Brain Surgery (Kindle edition). London: Weidenfeld & Nicolson; 2014, p. 210.
40 Womersley K, Ripullone K. How do we make feedback meaningful? BMJ. 2020; m17. doi:10.1136/bmj.m17
41 Miller A, Archer J. Impact of workplace based assessment on doctors' education and performance: A systematic review. BMJ. 2010; 341:c5064. doi:10.1136/bmj.c5064
42 Thaler RH, Sunstein CR. Nudge: Improving Decisions about Health, Wealth and Happiness. London: Penguin Books; 2009, p. 10.
43 Syed M. Black Box Thinking: Marginal Gains and the Secrets of High Performance. London: John Murray; 2015, p. 51.
44 Lloyd R. How Junior Doctors Think: A Guide for Reflective Practice [Internet]. Emergency Medical Journal Blog. 2016 October 19. Available from: https://stg-blogs.bmj.com/emj/2016/10/19/how-junior-doctors-think-a-guide-for-reflective-practice/
45 Francis R. The Mid Staffordshire NHS Foundation Trust Public Inquiry. 2013 February 6. Available from: https://commonslibrary.parliament.uk/research-briefings/sn06690/
46 Reason J. Doctor – Tell me the truth. BBC Radio 4; 2012. Available from: https://www.bbc.co.uk/sounds/play/b01cjm5d
47 Reason J. A Life in Error: From Little Slips to Big Disasters (Kindle edition). Farnham: Ashgate Publishing Limited; 2013, p. 74.
48 Reason J. Managing the Risks of Organizational Accidents. Aldershot: Ashgate Publishing Limited; 1997.

49 Davies A. Episode 45: Scott Weingart – Useful mental strategies of a thoughtful ED intensivist and hugely influential podcaster. [Internet]. Mastering Intensive Care. 2019 July 22. Available from: https://masteringintensivecare.libsyn.com/episode-45-scott-weingart-useful-mental-strategies-of-a-thoughtful-ed-intensivist-and-hugely-influential-podcaster

50 Jaye P, Thomas L, Reedy G. "The Diamond": A structure for simulation debrief. Clinical Teacher. 2015 May 25. 12; 171–5. doi:10.1111/tct.12300

51 Wu AW. Medical error: The second victim. BMJ. 2000; 320(7237): 726–7. doi:10.1136/bmj.320.7237.726

52 Davies A. Episode 21: Martin Bromiley – Turning tragedy into safer health-care with attention to human factors (DasSMACC special episode) [Internet]. Mastering Intensive Care. 2017 December 1. Available from: https://masteringintensivecare.libsyn.com/episode-21-martin-bromiley-turning-tragedy-into-safer-healthcare-by-attention-to-human-factors-dassmacc-special-episode

53 Reason J. A Life in Error: From Little Slips to Big Disasters (Kindle edition). Farnham: Ashgate Publishing Limited; 2013, p. 84.

Chapter 3: Healthy Safety

54 Reason J. A Life in Error: From Little Slips to Big Disasters (Kindle edition). Farnham: Ashgate Publishing Limited; 2013, p. 84.

55 Hollnagel E, Wears RL, Braithwaite J. From safety-I to safety-II: A white paper; 2010. Available from: https://www.england.nhs.uk/signuptosafety/wp-content/uploads/sites/16/2015/10/safety-1-safety-2-whte-papr.pdf

56 Thaler R. Misbehaving: The Making of Behavioural Economics. London: Penguin Books; 2016, p. 34.

57 Turner C. When Rudeness in Teams Turns Deadly [Internet]. London: TEDxExeter; 2019. Available from: https://www.tedxexeter.com/speakers/chris-turner-2/

58 Porath C. Mastering Civility: A Manifesto for the Workplace. New York: Grand Central Publishing; 2016.

59 Porath C, Pearson C. The price of incivility. Harvard Business Review Magazine. 2013 February. Available from: https://hbr.org/2013/01/the-price-of-incivility

60 Rosenstein AH, O'Daniel M. A survey of the impact of disruptive behaviors and communication defects on patient safety. Joint Commission Journal on Quality and Patient Safety. 2008; 34(8):464–71. doi:10.1016/s1553-7250(08)34058-6

61 Riskin A, Erez A, Foulk TA, Kugelman A, Gover A, Shoris I, et al. The impact of rudeness on medical team performance: A randomized trial. Pediatrics. 2015; 136(3):487–95. doi:10.1542/peds.2015-1385

62 Katz D, Blasius K, Isaak R, Lipps J, Kushelev M, Goldberg A, et al. Exposure to incivility hinders clinical performance in a simulated operative crisis. BMJ Qual Saf. 2019; 28(9):750–7. doi:10.1136/bmjqs-2019-009598

63 Cooper B, Giordano CR, Erez A, Foulk TA, Reed H, Berg KB. Trapped by a first hypothesis: How rudeness leads to anchoring. Journal of Applied Psychology. 2022; 107(3):481–502. doi:10.1037/apl0000914

64 Croskerry P. The importance of cognitive errors in diagnosis and strategies to minimize them. Academic Medicine. 2003; 78(8):775–80. doi:10.1097/00001888-200308000-00003

65 Watson C. The Courage to Care: A Call for Compassion. London: Vintage; 2020, pp. 198–9.

66 Edmondson AC. The Fearless Organisation: Creating Psychological Safety in the Workplace for Learning, Innovation and Growth. Hoboken, NJ: John Wiley & Sons, Inc.; 2019, pp. xvi–32.

67 Syed M. Black Box Thinking: Marginal Gains and the Secrets of High Performance. London: John Murray; 2015, p. 24.

68 Syed M. Black Box Thinking: Marginal Gains and the Secrets of High Performance. London: John Murray; 2015, p. 32.

69 Pronovost P, Vohr E. Safe Patients, Smart Hospitals: How One Doctor's Checklist Can Help Us Change Health Care from the Inside Out (Kindle edition). New York: Penguin Group (USA); 2010.

70 Pian-Smith MCM, Simon R, Minehart RD, Podraza M, Rudolph J, Walzer T, et al. Teaching residents the two-challenge rule: A simulation-based approach to improve education and patient safety. Simulation in Healthcare. 2009; 4(2):84–91. doi:10.1097/SIH.0b013e31818cffd3

71 Jayamohan J. Everything That Makes Us Human: Case Notes of a Children's Brain Surgeon (Kindle edition). London: Michael O'Mara Books Ltd; 2020, p. 77.

72 Lauria MJ, Gallo IA, Rush S, Brooks J, Spiegel R, Weingart SD. Psychological skills to improve emergency care providers' performance under stress. Ann Emerg Med. 2017; 70(6):884–90. doi:10.1016/j.annemergmed.2017.03.018
73 Shem S. The House of God (Black Swan edition). London: Transworld Publishers; 1985, p. 48.
74 Fredrickson B. Positivity: Discover the Upward Spiral That Will Change Your Life. New York: Crown Publishing Group; 2009.
75 Davies A. Episode 13: Sara Gray – Voices in my head (DasSMACC special episode) [Internet]. Mastering Intensive Care. 2017 August 16. Available from: https://masteringintensivecare.libsyn.com/episode-13-sara-gray-voices-in-my-head-dassmacc-special-episode
76 Letswaart M, Butler AJ, Jackson PL, Edwards MG. Editorial: Mental practice: Clinical and experimental research in imagery and action observation. Frontiers in Human Neuroscience. 2015. doi:10.3389/fnhum.2015.00573
77 Arora S, Aggarwal R, Sirimanna P, Moran A, Grantcharov T, Kneebone R, et al. Mental practice enhances surgical technical skills: A randomized controlled study. Ann Surg. 2011; 253(2):265–70. doi:10.1097/SLA.0b013e318207a789
78 Cragg J, Mushtaq F, Lal N, Garnham A, Hallissey M, Graham T, et al. Surgical cognitive simulation improves real-world surgical performance: Randomized study. BJS Open. 2021; 5(3). doi:10.1093/bjsopen/zrab003
79 Davies A. Mastering Intensive Care, Episode 15: Peter Brindley – Human factors including being a good person, listening well and tackling burnout (DasSMACC special episode) [Internet]. Mastering Intensive Care. 2017 August 30. Available from: https://masteringintensivecare.libsyn.com/episode-15-peter-brindley-human-factors-including-being-a-good-person-listening-well-and-tackling-burnout-dassmacc-special-episode

Chapter 4: Night Mode

80 Maggs F, Mallet M. Mortality in out-of-hours emergency medical admissions – More than just a weekend effect. Journal of the Royal College of Physicians of Edinburgh. 2010; 40(2):115–8. doi:10.4997/JRCPE.2010.205
81 British Medical Association. Fatigue and sleep deprivation – The impact of different working patterns on doctors. 2018. Available from:

https://www.bma.org.uk/media/1074/bma_fatigue-sleep-deprivation-briefing-jan2017.pdf

82 Landrigan CP, Rothschild JM, Cronin JW, Kaushal R, Burdick E, Katz JT, et al. Effect of reducing interns' work hours on serious medical errors in intensive care units. New England Journal of Medicine. 2004; 351(18):1838–48. doi:10.1056/NEJMoa041406

83 Folkard S, Tucker P. Shift work, safety and productivity. Occupational Medicine. 2003; 53:95–101. doi:10.1093/occmed/kqg047

84 van Dongen HPA, Maislin G, Mullington JM, Dinges DF. The cumulative cost of additional wakefulness: Dose-response effects on neurobehavioral functions and sleep physiology from chronic sleep restriction and total sleep deprivation. Sleep. 2003; 26(2):117–26. doi:10.1093/sleep/26.2.117

85 The Decision Lab. Why do we make worse decisions at the end of the day? [Internet]. TheDecisionLab.com. Available from: https://thedecisionlab.com/biases/decision-fatigue

86 Tierney J. Do you suffer from decision fatigue? New York Times Magazine. 2011 August 17. Available from: https://www.nytimes.com/2011/08/21/magazine/do-you-suffer-from-decision-fatigue.html

87 Allan JL, Johnston DW, Powell DJH, Farquharson B, Jones MC, Leckie G, et al. Clinical decisions and time since rest break: An analysis of decision fatigue in nurses. Health Psychology. 2019; 38(4):318–24. doi:10.1037/hea0000725

88 Spears D, Duh J, Geruso M, Gupta N, Haushofer J, Mullainathan S, et al. Economic decision-making in poverty depletes behavioral control [Internet]. B.E. Journal of Economic Analysis & Policy. 2011; 11. Available from: https://citeseerx.ist.psu.edu/viewdoc/download?doi=10.1.1.1080.299&rep=rep1&type=pdf

89 Lewis M. Obama's way. Vanity Fair. 2012 September 11. Available from: https://www.vanityfair.com/news/2012/10/michael-lewis-profile-barack-obama

90 Schwartz B. The Paradox of Choice: Why More Is Less (Kindle edition). London: Harper Collins e-books; 2007, p. 114.

91 Allan J, Powell D, Ferguson K, Plunkett E. Breaks at breaking point – Doctors need to take time out in a pandemic [Internet]. BMJ Opinion. 2020. Available from: https://blogs.bmj.com/bmj/2020/10/02/breaks-at-breaking-point-doctors-need-to-take-time-out-in-a-pandemic/

92 Park AE, Zahiri HR, Hallbeck MS, Augenstein V, Sutton E, Yu D, et al. Intraoperative "micro-breaks" with targeted stretching enhance surgeon physical function and mental focus a multicenter cohort study. Annals of Surgery. 2017; 265(2):340–6. doi:10.1097/SLA.0000000000001665

93 Engelmann C, Schneider M, Kirschbaum C, Grote G, Dingemann J, Schoof S, et al. Effects of intraoperative breaks on mental and somatic operator fatigue: A randomized clinical trial. Surgical Endoscopy. 2011; 25(4):1245–50. doi:10.1007/s00464-010-1350-1

94 Danziger S, Levav J, Avnaim-Pesso L. Extraneous factors in judicial decisions. Proceedings of the National Academy of Sciences of the United States of America. 2011; 108(17):6889–92. doi:10.1007/s00464-010-1350-1

95 Walker M. Why We Sleep: The New Science of Sleep and Dreams. London: Penguin Random House; 2018, p. 25.

96 Davies A. Episode 15: Peter Brindley – Human factors including being a good person, listening well and tackling burnout (DasSMACC special episode) [Internet]. Mastering Intensive Care. 2017 August 30. Available from: https://masteringintensivecare.libsyn.com/episode-15-peter-brindley-human-factors-including-being-a-good-person-listening-well-and-tackling-burnout-dassmacc-special-episode

97 Walker M. Why We Sleep: The New Science of Sleep and Dreams. London: Penguin Random House; 2018, p. 27.

98 McKenna H, Wilkes M. Optimising sleep for night shifts. BMJ. 2018; 360:j5637. doi:10.1136/bmj.j5637

99 Webb S. Exhausted doctor killed driving home from night shift when he 'fell asleep at the wheel.' Mirror Online [Internet]. 2016 July 12. Available from: https://www.mirror.co.uk/news/uk-news/exhausted-doctor-killed-driving-home-8402981

100 Tefft BC. Acute Sleep Deprivation and Risk of Motor Vehicle Crash Involvement [Internet]. Washington, DC. 2016. Available from: https://aaafoundation.org/acute-sleep-deprivation-risk-motor-vehicle-crash-involvement/

101 Walker M. Why We Sleep: The New Science of Sleep and Dreams. London: Penguin Random House; 2018, pp. 142–3.

102 McClelland L, Holland J, Lomas JP, Redfern N, Plunkett E. A national survey of the effects of fatigue on trainees in anaesthesia in the UK. Anaesthesia. 2017; 72(9):1069–77. doi:10.1111/anae.13965

103 McClelland L, Plunkett E, McCrossan R, Ferguson K, Fraser J, Gildersleve C, et al. A national survey of out-of-hours working and fatigue in consultants in anaesthesia and paediatric intensive care in the UK and Ireland. Anaesthesia. 2019; 74(12):1509–23. doi:10.1111/anae.14819

Interlude – Going Viral

104 Clarke R. Breathtaking: Inside the NHS in a Time of Pandemic (Kindle edition). London: Little, Brown; 2021.
105 Pimenta D. Duty of Care: One NHS Doctor's Story of Courage and Compassion on the COVID-19 Frontline (Kindle edition). London: Welbeck Non-Fiction Limited; 2020.
106 Calvert J, Arbuthnott G. Failures of State: The Inside Story of Britain's Battle with Coronavirus. London: Harper Collins; 2021.

Chapter 5: Their Final Doctor

107 Buckman R. How to Break Bad News: A Guide for Health Care Professionals. Baltimore: Johns Hopkins University Press; 1992.
108 Fecile J, Mars R. Episode 306: Breaking bad news [Internet]. 99 Percent Invisible. 2018 August 5. Available from: https://99percentinvisible.org/episode/breaking-bad-news/
109 Kübler-Ross E. On Death and Dying. (1st edition). New York: Macmillan Company; 1969.
110 Buckman R. I Don't Know What to Say. . .: How to Help and Support Someone Who Is Dying. New York: Vintage Books; 1989.
111 Baile WF, Buckman R, Lenzi R, Glober G, Beale EA, Kudelka AP. SPIKES – A six-step protocol for delivering bad news: Application to the patient with cancer. Oncologist. 2000; 5(4):302–11. doi:10.1634/theoncologist.5-4-302
112 Crowe L. Unravelling grief and loss [Internet]. Coda change. 2020. Available from: https://codachange.org/unravelling-grief-and-loss/
113 Murray J. Understanding Loss: A Guide for Caring for Those Facing Adversity. London: Routledge; 2015.
114 Morgan M. When nothing is the right thing to say. BMJ. 2020 February 18; 368:m574. doi:10.1136/bmj.m574

115 Clarke R. Dear Life: A Doctor's Story of Love and Loss (Kindle edition). London: Little, Brown; 2020, p. 194.

116 Mannix K. Listen: How to Find the Words for Tender Conversations. London: William Collins; 2021, p. 67.

117 Mannix K. Listen: How to Find the Words for Tender Conversations (Kindle edition). London: William Collins; 2021, p. 286.

118 Hobgood C, Harward D, Newton K, Davis W. The educational intervention "GRIEV_ING" improves the death notification skills of residents. Academic Emergency Medicine. 2005; 12(4):296–301. doi:10.1197/j.aem.2004.12.008

119 Hobgood CD, Tamayo-Sarver JH, Hollar DW, Hollar DW, Sawning S. GRIEV_ING: Death notification skills and applications for fourth-year medical students. Teaching and Learning in Medicine. 2009; 21(3):207–19. doi:10.1080/10401330903018445

120 Hobgood C, Mathew D, Woodyard DJ, Shofer FS, Brice JH. Death in the field: Teaching paramedics to deliver effective death notifications using the educational intervention "GRIEV-ING." Prehospital Emergency Care. 2013; 17(4):501–10. doi:10.3109/10903127.2013.804135

121 Mannix K. Listen: How to Find the Words for Tender Conversations (Kindle edition). London: William Collins; 2021, p. 142.

122 Obama B. A Promised Land. (1st edition). London: Viking; 2020, p. 379.

123 Rosen M. Many Different Kinds of Love: A Story of Life, Death and the NHS. London: Ebury Press; 2021.

124 NHS Education for Scotland. Dealing with bereavement in the workplace & staff wellbeing [Internet]. Support around Death. 2020. Available from: https://www.sad.scot.nhs.uk/covid-19/dealing-with-bereavement-in-the-workplace-staff-wellbeing/

125 Peterson JB. 12 Rules for Life: An Antidote to Chaos. London: Allen Lane; 2018.

126 Neighbour R. The Inner Consultation: How to Develop an Effective and Intuitive Consulting Style. (2nd edition). Oxford: Radcliffe Publishing; 2005, pp. 211–27.

127 Walton M. Processing Trauma: Resilience may not lie within individuals, but between individuals [Internet]. BMJ Opinion. 2018 May 15. Available from: https://blogs.bmj.com/bmj/2018/05/15/processing-trauma-resilience-may-not-lie-within-individuals-but-between-individuals/

128 Walton M. Resilience – One Team's Trauma [Internet]. United Kingdom: YouTube; 2018 May 16. Available from: https://www.youtube.com/watch?v=DY60ZOWBvDc

Chapter 6: Clinging to the Raft

129 Berger J, Mohr J. A Fortunate Man: The Story of a Country Doctor. Edinburgh: Canongate Books Ltd; 2016.
130 Francis G. John Berger's A fortunate man: A masterpiece of witness. Guardian [Internet]. 2015 Feb 7. Available from: https://www.theguardian.com/books/2015/feb/07/john-sassall-country-doctor-a-fortunate-man-john-berger-jean-mohr
131 Shem S. The House of God (Black Swan edition). London: Transworld Publishers; 1985, p. 289.
132 Gerada C. Beneath the White Coat: Doctors, Their Minds and Mental Health (Kindle edition). Abingdon: Routledge; 2021
133 Vedantam S. Between two worlds [Internet]. Hidden Brain. 2020 November 9. Available from: https://hiddenbrain.org/podcast/between-two-worlds/
134 Watson C. The Language of Kindness: A Nurse's Story (Vintage edition). London: Penguin Random House; 2019, p. 125.
135 Worthy L, Lavigne T, Romero F. Culture and Psychology: How People Shape and Are Shaped by Culture. Phoenix, AZ: Pressbooks; 2020, p. 324. Available from: https://open.maricopa.edu/culturepsychology/
136 Conner KO. What is code-switching? Understanding the impact of code-switching for racial and ethnic minorities. Psychology Today [Internet]. 2020 December 3. Available from: https://www.psychologytoday.com/us/blog/achieving-health-equity/202012/what-is-code-switching
137 Morton JM. Cultural code-switching: Straddling the achievement gap. Journal of Political Philosophy. 2014; 22(3):259–81. doi:10.1111/jopp.12019
138 Austen L. Increasing emotional support for healthcare workers can rebalance clinical detachment and empathy. British Journal of General Practice. 2016; 66(648):376–7. doi:10.3399/bjgp16X685957
139 Halpern J. What is clinical empathy? J Gen Intern Med. 2003; 18(8):670–4. doi:10.1046/j.1525-1497.2003.21017.x

140 Richardson R. A necessary inhumanity? Med Humanit. 2000; 26(2):104–6. doi:10.1136/mh.26.2.104
141 Osler W. Aequanimitas. London: Ravenio Books; 1927.
142 Böckers A, Jerg-Bretzke L, Lamp C, Brinkmann A, Traue HC, Böckers TM. The gross anatomy course: An analysis of its importance. Anat Sci Educ. 2010; 3(1):3–11. doi:10.1002/ase.124
143 Hildebrandt S. Developing empathy and clinical detachment during the dissection course in gross anatomy. Anat Sci Educ. 2010; 3(4):216. doi:10.1002/ase.145
144 Coulehan J, Granek IA. Commentary: "I hope I'll continue to grow": Rubrics and reflective writing in medical education. Academic Medicine. 2012; 87(1):8–10. doi:10.1097/ACM.0b013e31823a98ba
145 Awdish R. In Shock: How Nearly Dying Made Me a Better Intensive Care Doctor. London: Bantam Press; 2018, pp. 164–5.
146 Awdish R. Bio [Internet]. 2017. Available from: https://www.ranaawdishmd.com/bio
147 Goodrich J. Supporting hospital staff to provide compassionate care: Do Schwartz Center Rounds work in English hospitals? J R Soc Med. 2012; 105(3):117–22. doi:10.1258/jrsm.2011.110183
148 Maben J, Taylor C, Dawson J, Leamy M, McCarthy I, Reynolds E, et al. A realist informed mixed-methods evaluation of Schwartz Center Rounds® in England. Health Services and Delivery Research. 2018; 6(37):1–260. doi:10.3310/hsdr06370
149 Brown B. Daring Greatly: How the Courage to Be Vulnerable Transforms the Way We Live, Love, Parent, and Lead (Kindle edition). London: Penguin; 2013, p. 137.
150 Neighbour R. Detachment and empathy. British Journal of General Practice. 2016; 66(650):460. doi:10.3399/bjgp16X686737
151 Neighbour R. The Inner Consultation: How to Develop an Effective and Intuitive Consulting Style. Oxford: Radcliffe Publishing; 2005, p. 203.
152 Neighbour R. The Inner Physician: Why and How to Practise "Big Picture Medicine." London: The Royal College of General Practitioners; 2016, pp. 212–14.
153 Crichton M. Travels. London: Pan; 1989.
154 Forster E. Howards End. London: Penguin Books; 2000.

155 British Medical Association. Moral distress and moral injury: Recognising and tackling it for UK doctors. 2021 June. Available from: https://www.bma.org.uk/media/4209/bma-moral-distress-injury-survey-report-june-2021.pdf
156 Mealer M, Moss M. Moral distress in ICU nurses. Intensive Care Med. 2016; 42(10):1615–7. doi:10.1007/s00134-016-4441-1
157 Cannon J. Breaking and Mending: A Junior Doctor's Stories of Compassion & Burnout. London: Profile Books Limited; 2019, p.103.
158 Segal F. Mother Ship. London: Chatto & Windus; 2019, p. 152.
159 Kalanithi P. When Breath Becomes Air. London: Vintage Digital; 2016, pp. 60–1.
160 Dunbar RIM. Neocortex size as a constraint on group size in primates. J Hum Evol. 1992; 22(6):469–93. doi:10.1016/0047-2484(92)90081-J
161 Hill RA, Dunbar RIM. Social network size in humans. Human Nature. 2003; 14(1):53–72. doi:10.1007/s12110-003-1016-y
162 Krotoski A. Robin Dunbar: We can only ever have 150 friends at most. Guardian [Internet]. 2010 March 14. Available from: https://www.theguardian.com/technology/2010/mar/14/my-bright-idea-robin-dunbar
163 Morton JM. Moving Up Without Losing Your Way: The Ethical Costs of Upward Mobility. Woodstock: Princeton University Press; 2019, p. 26.
164 Coles R. The Madness of Grief: A Memoir of Love and Loss (Kindle edition). London: Weidenfeld & Nicolson; 2021, p. 108.

Chapter 7: Sliding Hospital Doors

165 The General Medical Council. GMC approved postgraduate curricula [Internet]. Available from: https://www.gmc-uk.org/education/standards-guidance-and-curricula/curricula
166 Oishi LN. Enhancing Career Development Agency in Emerging Adulthood: An Intervention Using Design Thinking [Internet]. Stanford University; 2012. Available from: https://purl.stanford.edu/tt351qn0806
167 Reilly TS. Designing Life: Studies of Emerging Adult Development [Internet]. Stanford University; 2013. Available from: https://stacks.stanford.edu/file/druid:xt225kd5463/Reilly%20Thesis%204-24-augmented.pdf

168 Burnett B, Evans D. Designing Your Life: Build the Perfect Career, Step by Step. London: Penguin Random House UK; 2018.
169 Burnett B, Evans D. Designing Your Life: Build the Perfect Career, Step by Step. London: Penguin Random House UK; 2016, p. 8.
170 Eldon K, Eldon D. The journey is the destination: The Journals of Dan Eldon. San Francisco: Chronicle Books; 2017.
171 Kay A. This Is Going to Hurt: Secret Diaries of a Junior Doctor. London: Picador; 2017, p. 61.
172 Kalanithi P. When Breath Becomes Air (Kindle edition). London: Vintage Digital; 2016, p. 53.
173 Burnett B, Evans D. Designing Your Life: Build the Perfect Career, Step by Step. London: Penguin Random House UK; 2016, p. 38.
174 Burnett B, Evans D. Designing Your Life: Build the Perfect Career, Step by Step. London: Penguin Random House UK; 2016, p. 79.
175 Burnett B, Evans D. Designing Your Life: Build the Perfect Career, Step by Step. London: Penguin Random House UK; 2016, p. 79.
176 Hesse H. The Glass Bead Game. Vintage Books. London: Penguin Random House UK; 2000.
177 Haig M. The Midnight Library (Digital edition). Edinburgh: Canongate Books; 2020.
178 Haig M. The Midnight Library (Digital edition). Edinburgh: Canongate Books; 2020, p. 175.
179 Haig M. The Midnight Library (Digital edition). Edinburgh: Canongate Books; 2020, p. 273.
180 Haig M. The Midnight Library (Digital edition). Edinburgh: Canongate Books; 2020, p. 280.
181 Skopeliti C. UK's number of doctors per capita is one of lowest in Europe. Guardian [Internet]. 2019 December 23. Available from: https://www.theguardian.com/society/2019/dec/23/uk-has-second-lowest-number-of-doctors-per-capita-in-europe
182 Dubner SJ. The upside of quitting [Internet]. Freakonomics Radio. 2011 September 30. Available from: https://freakonomics.com/podcast/the-upside-of-quitting-3/
183 Schwartz B. The Paradox of Choice: Why More Is Less (Kindle edition). London: Harper Collins e-books; 2007, p. 122.

184 BMJ. Sharp scratch: Leaving medicine. BMJ Talk Medicine. 2020. Available from: https://soundcloud.com/bmjpodcasts/leaving-medicine

185 Vedantam S. Loss and renewal [Internet]. Hidden Brain. 2020 August 17. Available from: https://hiddenbrain.org/podcast/you-2-0-loss-and-renewal/

Conclusion – It's About Time

186 Hunt J. Zero: Eliminating Unnecessary Deaths in a Post-pandemic NHS (Kindle edition). London: Swift Press; 2022, p. 249.

187 Groopman J. How Doctors Think (First Mariner Books edition). Boston: Houghton Mifflin Company; 2008, p. 36.

188 Vedantam S. Think fast with Daniel Kahneman [Internet]. Hidden Brain. 2018 March 13. Available from: https://hiddenbrain.org/podcast/think-fast-with-daniel-kahneman/

189 Dworkis D. The Emergency Mind (Kindle Edition). Los Angeles: Sangfroid Press; 2021, p. 159.

190 Rilke RM, Herter Norton MD. Letters to a Young Poet (Revised edition). London: W. W. Norton & Company; 1993, p. 54.

INDEX

Note: Page numbers in *italic* indicate a figure and page numbers in **bold** indicate a table on the corresponding page.

Printed in the United States
by Baker & Taylor Publisher Services